ONE WOMAN'S PURSUIT OF HAPPINESS
IN THE FACE OF CHRONIC ILLNESS

EVERYTHING

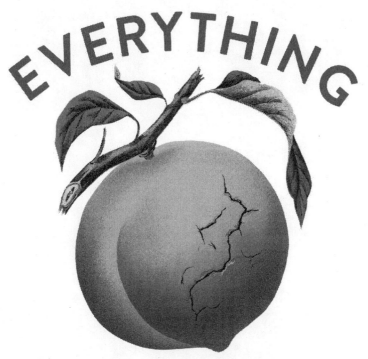

IS NOT
PEACHEY

LISA PEACHEY

This book is dedicated to my parents.

To my mother, whose kindness, care, and thoughtfulness were matched only by her playful spirit. She always put her children first, striving to do right by us with unwavering love. Her warmth touched everyone fortunate enough to know her, and her absence is deeply felt by all. I cherish every memory and am grateful for every moment we shared.

To my dad, affectionately known as Bobarino, who continues to fill my life with laughter and steadfast support. Even when my choices, ambitions, or goals baffle him, he stands by me, offering encouragement that knows no bounds. I wouldn't trade him for anything in the world.

Mom and Dad, my love for you both is eternal.

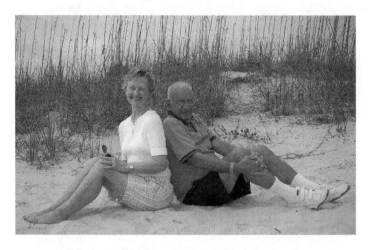

Mom and Dad on their 50th wedding anniversary vacation in Florida.

CONTENTS

INTRODUCTION

I had always thought of myself as a healthy person. Yes, I have struggled with my weight off and on for as long as I can remember, and I have never been what would be considered athletic. In general, though, I had been free of afflictions for most of my life, had excellent eyesight, felt pretty good, and considered myself normal.

Until I wasn't.

Chronic illness creeps up on you. You know you are healthy when you *don't* notice your well-being, or lack thereof, or are aware of what your body is doing every day. Sure, there are good days and bad days. Maybe one day, you didn't get quite enough sleep, or you had a hangover or a bit of a cold, so you are aware that you don't feel so good at that moment. Other times, you really enjoyed going to the gym, or maybe you went for an extra-long walk and felt great afterward. You notice your body but more in an afterthought kind of way.

It's kind of like our teeth. We rarely think about them other than basic maintenance like brushing and flossing. But when you have a toothache, suddenly, your whole world revolves around your teeth, and you are very aware of every tooth in your mouth, every bite of food, or the temperature of any liquid. Ice cream is too cold and becomes a distant memory. Crunchy food is challenging, and you suddenly realize you've been chewing exclusively on one side of your mouth for a while and can't recall when that started.

Our health is like that: we don't notice it much, even as we start to slide down that slippery slope with the occasional small problem. You can ignore one or two symptoms, especially if they seem random or explainable and don't interfere too much with your life. Then there are a few more, and maybe you think you're having a bad winter or just getting older. Slowly these issues add up and begin to impact your daily routine.

One day, seemingly abruptly, you are living a completely different life. Every waking moment revolves around managing your body with all of its particular needs and requirements, and you wonder how you got there and if you will ever get back to the way it was before.

This is my story. I am not a doctor or a medical professional, and this book is not intended to be medical advice or replace the care of a doctor. I repeat: I am not giving medical advice. I am simply telling my story and sharing my experiences and observations.

My intention is to get people to question things—in fact, everything. I have spent so much of my life allowing authority figures to dictate what was appropriate or safe for me, and I let them tell me how to proceed when things went wrong. I trusted them, and that trust was broken. Now, I know better and feel compelled to relate what I have learned. I hope that by sharing the story of my journey, I can help other chronically ill people find a path forward for themselves and hopefully even prevent others from becoming sick.

This book is also for anyone who has chronically ill people in their lives who they don't know how to help. Because our symptoms are so often intangible to everyone around us, it's easy for us to be labeled as hypochondriacs. Perhaps this book could at least give a friend or family member some understanding of what we are going through and how they could help—without us having to ask. Believe it or not, most of us *hate* to ask. We really just want to be normal.

CHAPTER 1

WALK A MILE IN MY SHOES PLEASE...

I'm an environmentally ill, chemically sensitive person living in the toxic landscape that is our modern world.

But what does that really mean? Allow me to share a glimpse of my life to provide insight into the reality of living with chronic illness. There are times when I long to do the simple things that others take for granted, to feel normal, and I find myself going to great lengths to pretend that I can.

For those of us who are chemically sensitive, asthmatic, or need to avoid fragrances and chemicals, even the thought of travel can be overwhelming. What should be a simple pleasure becomes a daunting, often exhausting task fraught with challenges others might never consider. Whether it's a necessary trip for medical treatment, business, or a much-needed vacation, the journey is anything but straightforward. Every step of the process—from packing to navigating public spaces—requires meticulous planning and constant vigilance. There are many obstacles, and the stakes are high, turning what should be an exciting adventure into a stressful ordeal. What if you just simply want to go on vacation?

• • •

It's winter in Massachusetts, the slow season for your business, so you can finally take some time off and go on vacation - someplace tropical. You can almost feel the sun's warmth on your skin and the sand between your toes. What are you waiting for? Just hop onto the internet and book a trip for yourself, right?

Not so fast hotshot - you are facing a multitude of obstacles.

No matter where you go, you will need to pack your clothes, so what are you using for luggage? Does it smell like nothing, or did it absorb odors and chemicals from the airplanes, hotels, etc., of previous trips? These places routinely spray chemicals for all kinds of reasons, including insect control, cleaning, and what they call – deodorizing, all of which tend to contaminate luggage.

It's challenging at best, and sometimes impossible, to remove these contaminants, so if you need new luggage, which tends to be chemically offensive, did you think about buying it months ago to let it off-gas its new smell somewhere out of your living space? Even then, it probably still somewhat stinks like chemicals. In the worst-case scenario, you line your suitcases with bath towels, hoping your clothes won't pick up those contaminants.

Have you decided on a destination? Maybe you read that the best beaches in the world are in Turks and Caicos, and you are daydreaming about that famous baby powder white and pink sand. So you start looking, but there are no direct flights from Boston to Turks and Caicos. You would have to change planes no matter what. Are you up for that? Traveling is difficult enough because of your sensitivities. Are you willing to suffer through that extra leg of travel? I didn't think so.

You run into a similar problem with many Caribbean islands. Hawaii and the South Pacific are, of course, out of the question. After extensive research, you narrow down a list of tropical destinations you can reach in a nonstop flight from Boston. You decide on Aruba.

Now, all you need to do is find lodging. Will you stay in a hotel, a resort, or an Airbnb? Of course, you must make countless phone calls and send many emails to find one that uses fragrance-free laundry products. Responses are sporadic, and often, the people you are corresponding with either clearly don't know what is being used at their property, or worse, they are just obviously telling you what you want to hear. Your excitement at deciding on your destination starts to wane as you repeatedly come up empty.

Experience has taught you the hard way that it's not an option for the establishment to just wash the sheets in fragrance-free detergent before your arrival. Scented laundry products infiltrate all textiles in a room, generally at a level that makes them toxic to you indefinitely, even if the sheets are washed in "free & clear" before your arrival. These products do not just wash out; they are designed to be *sticky* and are almost impossible to eliminate. And it's not just the linens that are the problem. Mattresses, furniture, carpet, drapes, all the textiles, and soft or porous surfaces will have absorbed these chemicals, making the room a toxic soup that is uninhabitable to you. You need to stay somewhere that only uses fragrance-free laundry products all the time, and ideally has no carpet in the room, just to have a fighting chance of not getting sick.

You struck out with Aruba, so it's back to the drawing board. Finally, you find a resort in Puerto Rico that can confirm they use fragrance-free laundry products. Now you can book a flight.

Can you afford a first-class ticket so you'll have more space around you with less chance of secondhand fragrance from the other passengers? If you are going to be in the main cabin, it will be a very problematic and miserable flight. Passengers in first class also tend to have more access to the flight attendants, so if you have special needs or requests, you are more likely to have better results. Also, you will be the first to deplane, which will get you the hell off the plane faster. You will be so desperate for clean air to breathe by the time the plane lands that you are ready to commit murder.

On the other hand, you don't want to sit too close to the lavatory, which can contain offensive chemicals. The exact location of your seat needs to be a very strategic decision.

What if there is no first-class or you can't afford it? Are you traveling alone or with a companion? When you are crammed in like sardines in the main cabin, how do you keep a safe bubble of personal space around you? You need to buy at least the seat next to you and hope that the person sitting in front of you doesn't have hair spray on or worse.

If the airline doesn't have first class, you can try to buy a seat in the first row so you won't have people in front of you, but you will be very close to the lavatory. Is that better than having someone with hairspray recline their seat so the back of their head is right in your face? How do you choose? You would never buy a ticket on an airline that does not allow you to choose your seat in advance; that would be a nightmare.

Finally, you book a flight. The good news is that this has turned into a family vacation, and you, your spouse, parents, in-laws, and other assorted family members are all going together. Everyone is excited about this trip because they know it is a big deal for you to make this happen. You bought main cabin tickets because you could select your seats and surround yourself with your family, building a bubble to buffer you from the other passengers. Problem solved.

The day of the trip arrives. Everyone else is super excited, but *your* anxiety is through the roof. You hope and pray that you will get through this day without too much pain and discomfort. You are determined not to be difficult and ruin the trip for your spouse or your family. You are quiet and subdued as you arrive at the airport.

You need to check in two hours before your flight departs. That means, once you've gotten through security, you will be trapped in the terminal waiting to board with hordes of people covered in every personal product imaginable. Your extended family is arriving separately, and they are running late. Do you set up camp at your gate, which is guaranteed to get very crowded in the hour before boarding? You will be back-to-back or next to people with laundry, hair spray, perfume, deodorant, after-shave, and more for the whole time.

It may be best to find an uncrowded spot away from the gate and other people, but will you then be the last one to board and have to stand in line forever with all of these people? You pray that your flight is on time and that boarding will go quickly and smoothly.

Eventually, your family arrives, and you allow yourself to be distracted by them. They are all happy and full of anticipation about the fabulous trip we have planned. You secretly are jealous that they have no anxiety or concerns about any part of this trip, only happy expectations.

Boarding goes quickly and without incident, and you settle in for the flight. With your family sitting all around you on the plane, you are somewhat insulated from the other passengers, and the flight is more or less without incident. The plane smells like cleaning products and bug spray, but thankfully, it's only a four-hour flight, so you get through it with just a headache and some brain fog.

After you arrive at your destination, how are you getting to your lodgings, and how far away is that? You can't just rent a car from Budget, Avis, or any of the usual car rental companies because they spray their cars with fragrance as part of the cleaning process.

If you are renting from a private car company (much more expensive), you can probably negotiate with them to provide you with a vehicle that has not been sprayed with fragrance and also isn't brand new and still off-gassing new-car chemicals. It will likely have leather seats that have had ArmorAll applied, so hopefully, you can tolerate that. Or you could use an app-based car service. Can you request a fragrance-free Uber or Lyft driver? Taxis are a treacherous last resort, but on this trip it's your best option from the airport.

You finally arrive at your resort, and it's the moment of truth. Is this room fragrance-free or not? You instantly identify that even though the linens have actually been washed in fragrance-free products, there is new wall-to-wall carpeting in the bedroom that was not in the photos online. You are horrified because carpet off-gasses formaldehyde, which is one of your triggers. On top of that, they used something super scented to "freshen" the carpet, so the room is most definitely *not* fragrance-free.

You don't want to ruin anyone else's trip by making a big deal. You can always drag some bedding into the bathroom and sleep on the tile floor. Hopefully, you are not going to spend a lot of time in your room anyway. You think this is still salvageable, and since your only other option is to find alternate lodging or go home, you decide to try to stick it out. Perhaps it just smells overwhelming because you have been traveling and inundated with toxic exposures all day. Maybe you just need some fresh air.

You are desperate to get out of your room, go for a swim, and get some sun. It's just early afternoon, so the day is not entirely ruined by travel. The pool is too heavily chlorinated for you, so your option is the beach. Of course, you can't wear most sunblock, but maybe you found one that won't make you sick. Now, you need to find a spot on the beach that is nowhere near anyone who might be spraying sunblock on themselves. You need to strategically place yourself upwind of anyone who might do that. Your family is being incredibly patient and non-judgmental. They let you steer this ship.

Finally, you relax and have a fabulous afternoon at the beach. You soak up the sun and feel the sand between your toes just like you dreamed of. You look forward to dinner. Hopefully, your server and nearby diners will be fragrance-free. Did you review the menu for this place beforehand to see if they had any food you could eat? Like most chronically ill people you have a number of food restrictions.

They have an extensive menu at dinner, and your family members are all quite pleased. But for you, as a vegan who doesn't eat gluten, your only option is a plain baked potato and a salad with just oil and vinegar. Fortunately, they have avocados in the kitchen, which you can get them to serve with your baked potato instead of sour cream.

It's depressing to have such limited dining options when you are on vacation. Still, you probably also factored that into your initial research of where you were going and know there is at least one restaurant nearby with interesting menu options that don't break any of your food rules. Tonight, you're too tired to find it and don't want to inconvenience your family. So you quietly eat your baked potato and salad even though it looks like it came from a high school cafeteria compared to the extravagant dinners served to everyone else.

There is an exciting show at the resort theater later that everyone wants to see, but after the torture of traveling, you just can't face being in close proximity to other people. What if they just cleaned the floors at the theater? After all of the day's exposures and triggers, you don't feel very well by now, so you return to your room to try to make the best of it.

Somehow though, the room seems even worse now than when you arrived. How did you not notice this earlier? You were probably in olfactory overload from the exposures at the airport and then the taxi ride to the resort. Even sleeping on the bathroom floor is no longer an option, as every surface seems to have been wiped down with scented cleaning products.

There is no way you can stay here. But you are already in Puerto Rico, and your family is here because *you* chose this place. You get on the internet and start looking at other lodging options; you can move to another resort or hotel – without uprooting your family.

You find a hotel nearby that might be better, so you decide to take a leap of faith and try it. They make promises to you on the phone about their rooms being fragrance-free. You move, leaving your family at the first hotel; not the worst-case scenario, but still not optimal. Upon arrival, you find plenty of cleaning product smells there too, but maybe it's not as bad as the other resort. You try to suck it up and power through, and at first, it seems like it will be okay because it has a slider facing the ocean, so you think you could just leave it open all night and get fresh air from the sea. But the pool is just a few floors down, and the chlorine and chemical smells wafting in are too much.

You have now started to become very symptomatic and realize that if you stay here much longer, the physical price may be higher than what you can afford. As much as you had been looking forward to this vacation, you realize it's time to pull the plug.

You spend the final wee hours of the morning on the internet booking a flight home. Defeated, as the sun rises, you arrange a car to take you to the airport. You leave your spouse, in-laws, and the rest of your family there to enjoy the vacation you selected and arranged – without you. Struggling physically, mentally, and emotionally, you fly home alone to get back to your safe bubble. You had hoped that this time it would be fun to go on a trip; you could be a tourist, a traveler even, and relax with the people you love. You had forgotten how impossible it can be. Will you ever be able to go anywhere again?

• • •

These experiences have actually happened to me. Although some of the locations have been changed for continuity, this is an aggregation of actual events in my life. I took that flight home, leaving my husband and our family behind. Lonely does not even remotely describe how I felt on that flight. Somehow, this is what my life had turned into. How did it get to this point? And more importantly, what did I do next?

CHAPTER 2

DID IT START BEFORE I WAS BORN?

I was born in Boston, Massachusetts, in 1965. My father was the only child of Italian immigrants, and my mother was one of five daughters born to Irish immigrants. In those days, the Irish and the Italians did not mix in Boston.

My Irish grandmother was, for all purposes, a single mom. Nana worked tirelessly, cleaning houses and raising five daughters on her own. She had no car, no family to help her, and a husband who spent most of his time and money in bars, occasionally showing up to wreak havoc. She took the bus to her many jobs, bringing my mom and aunts with her when they were too young for school. They didn't always know where their next meal was coming from.

My Italian grandfather worked in road construction and even lost a finger building a new highway, where today hundreds of thousands drive over its burial ground under Route 128, south of Boston. My Italian grandmother, Francesca, was a determined woman who worked at a shoe factory among mostly Irish laborers. She told everyone her name was Frances because she thought it sounded more American, and when they found out that her birthday was on Saint Patrick's Day, they loved her, and she had friends for life.

Growing up, I remember how everyone thought it was so funny that Grandma was born on Saint Patrick's Day; we'd always make a big deal of it and celebrate her birthday with lots of green and shamrocks. It wasn't until she died at age seventy-seven that my grandfather revealed she had been lying about her birthday. He set the record straight because he thought her death certificate should be correct. Even my dad never knew that she had made it up so that her Irish coworkers would accept her. No one alive remembers her actual birth date now.

My grandmother proved that people will generally accept something as fact if you say it with conviction and stick with it, even if it seems odd, unexpected, or unusual.

Despite the friction and animosity between the two cultures in Boston, my parents' marriage was supported by my Italian grandparents and my Irish grandmother. My Irish grandfather occasionally made a surprise appearance to voice his disapproval but was otherwise not a factor. Nana was happy to see her daughter marry a hardworking Catholic, and my Italian grandparents got the daughter they always wanted. Everyone was happy.

Everyone also wanted babies. Five long years went by. When my mom finally became pregnant with my older brother, the whole family rejoiced. Her doctor prescribed a drug called diethylstilbestrol (DES) and said it would prevent miscarriage. This was 1964.

It had been widely known in the medical world since the 1950s that DES (diethylstilbestrol) was proven to be not only ineffective for this purpose but, in fact, had been shown to cause miscarriage, as well as prenatal drug-induced cancer and/ or birth defects. It was such a problem that in 1971, the FDA had to ban its use during pregnancy because doctors were still prescribing it.

Mom's doctor not only prescribed DES along with strict bed rest for the entire pregnancy, he instructed her to drink plenty of alcohol and smoke cigarettes every day for relaxation. Naturally, she wanted to do everything possible to have a healthy baby. She trusted her doctor and did what she was told, never thinking to question. Despite a difficult pregnancy and this doctor's obvious negligence, my older brother miraculously managed to be born without complications. My parents and grandparents were ecstatic to finally have a baby and lavished attention on him. My mother was told she would never be able to conceive again.

Two months later, my mom became pregnant with me. Surprise! The same doctor, based on the "success" of DES with my brother, prescribed it again. Once more, she was told: strict bed rest, watch television, drink plenty of booze, and smoke cigarettes to stay calm. It boggles the mind now, but a doctor's word was law. My parents had been taught not to question authority, and this doctor was running the show.

Mom's pregnancy with me was even more difficult., She once again followed all the doctor's orders, *despite* which I somehow managed to be born. I was premature, only five pounds, but seemingly without a defect. (Although, I must have been desperate for a beer and a smoke right out of the womb, which would explain a few things.) The doctor told my parents to hurry up and take me home; if I pooped, I might be under the five-pound minimum weight for discharge.

My parents brought me home to the two-family house that my Italian grandparents owned in Boston. We lived on the second floor with Grandma and Grandpa downstairs. The focus of the entire household became getting Lisa to gain weight.

According to the data from the National Survey of Family Growth published in 1979, from 1961-1965, only 38% of women were breastfeeding for any duration, and only 12% were breastfeeding for three months or more.

My mother told me it was not only considered old-fashioned, low-class, and even disgusting, but the doctor told her that formulas were more nutritious than breast milk. I was an underweight baby; he said it was critical they provide me with the best modern formula. However, I had zero tolerance for the standard formula and refused to take it or keep it down from day one. The doctor, in his infinite wisdom, prescribed a *meat-based* formula for me. I can't believe that even existed. I don't know if he provided a recipe to whip up at home or if it was an obscure product available for a hot minute in the heyday of baby formula development. My mom told me it was pink, smelled awful, and disgusted her. Baby Me managed to choke it down long enough to survive to the age of being able to eat real food.

Family lore says I cried more than any other baby anyone knew, apparently in the history of the world. I wailed so often that neighbors would call and ask what was wrong with me. I wonder now if, in addition to my gruesome diet of meat milk, I was experiencing some kind of withdrawal from the substances I absorbed prenatally due to the doctor's prescription for a "healthy" pregnancy.

My early years were spent with my well-intentioned family doing their best to fatten me up. My Italian grandfather had a huge garden. He grew his own vegetables, including tomatoes, which he would make into tomato sauce. (They called it gravy, *not* sauce). Grandpa was an excellent cook, more so than my grandmother, who once added orange peel to a lasagna, making it inedible. Grandpa would make a big family dinner every Sunday. There was always pasta, sausages, meatballs with his homemade gravy, and other Italian specialties, taking advantage of what was in season in his garden. We all drank his homemade wine with meals, even the kids - for whom it was not watered down; my grandfather would be horrified by the insult to his wine if it was suggested.

Because of Grandpa's garden, we ate only fresh produce in the summer and fall, especially tomatoes. He had brought seeds from Italy, and his garden was a masterclass in how to produce the perfect tomato. As kids, we'd follow him around, and he would give us tomatoes to eat as if they were apples. If my mom wanted store-bought tomatoes in the winter, she would hide them because he found them to be an offense to his very purpose in life.

It wasn't until I was an adult and Grandpa was long gone, that I realized his tomatoes were truly exceptional. I have spent decades tasting heirlooms from farmer's markets, growing different varieties of tomatoes in backyard gardens and in pots, trying to identify a variety that would at least come close to what he grew.

I never appreciated what we had when we were young. Despite all the fresh produce and homemade food, as a child, what I really always wanted was Grandma's orange soda and cheesy poofs. Grandma's orange soda was always flat, and her cheesy poofs were always stale, and I loved that shit! It was like a neon orange extravaganza. You'd bite into a poof, and it wouldn't crunch; it would squish, and if you applied pressure on them in your mouth precisely the right way, you could even make them squeak. To this day, I live for all things orange, and when I say orange, I'm specifically thinking of that neon color of orange soda and cheesy poofs. It's all tied up in my head with memories of my grandmother, whom I adored.

My older brother liked the sweet stuff and loaded up on her candy and grape soda, which was always slightly fermented. I think she would wait for a sale and then lay in such a big supply of soda and snacks that everything would be stale by the time we consumed it. We didn't know the difference, we only knew that we were having special treats that our parents would never let us have. Grandma's pantry was in a league of its own for unhealthy snacks, weird mystery candy, and sugary drinks.

It occurs to me now that Grandpa never touched any of that stuff. While we kids were stuffing ourselves on stale neon junk, Grandpa would snack on fresh vegetables or fruit that he grew himself. He was healthy as a horse right up until the end. He literally was still shoveling snow off of his roof well into his late eighties until my dad put a stop to it.

Even though Grandpa was an excellent role model, showing us how to eat a healthy, organic, well-balanced whole-food diet, I spent the young years of my life developing unhealthy food addictions and eating habits. Because I had started as such a small and underweight baby, everyone habitually watched what I ate and always encouraged me to eat more. If I had second or third helpings, and make no mistake, they were counting and cheering me on, I would be praised for having a healthy appetite. There was *substantial* positive reinforcement given to both my brother and I if we overate – especially me, at a very unhealthy level.

My baby brother was born three days before my fifth birthday. My parents had twice been told my mother would never conceive again, so they referred to him as their "miracle baby." Fortunately, his birth took some of the focus off me, but for many years there was still an abundance of pressure always to have second and third helpings at Sunday dinner.

I was a fearful child with zero self-confidence, so I did what I was told. I announced I did not want to eat meat - animals were my friends. When my family reacted in horror, I quickly backed down. I know they loved me and meant well, so I have never blamed them, but my lifelong struggle with my relationship with food has been an issue not easily overcome.

Over the years, my mother made many notes in my baby book about my eating habits and how I interacted with my brothers - the usual stuff. Most notable is Mom's repeated use of the word "fussy" in relation to my - pretty much everything. Nearly every entry includes a comment about me being "fussy" for the first six years of my life. It was the word she used to describe me in general, as I think she did not want to classify me as *unhappy*, but she knew something was…off.

Mom noticed I was a little chubby as I slid into my tween years, recording "still eating too much and really too heavy." I think Mom was starting to struggle at that point with what my grandmother was feeding me on the sly. Until then, weight was not something I had thought about or even had much self-awareness about. But as a tween, that was starting to change.

Around the same time, I once again informed my family that I did not want to eat animals anymore, and once again, I was met with a lot of resistance. We had moved to our own house in the suburbs outside of Boston, so although the dynamic was a little different without my grandparents living just downstairs, we still had Sunday dinners with them, which meant we had two days of leftovers. Pasta, meatballs, sausages, etc., were on the menu for us three days a week well into my teens. My parents had a very traditional view of what our meals were supposed to look like, and I was expected to appreciate that we had food on the table and not question what it was or where it came from.

My response to this was not eating. I went from being a chubby child to an overly thin teenager, flirting with anorexia. I didn't want to eat meat at all. Also, I knew now that being thin was desirable; my "solution" seemed obvious and uncomplicated. Naturally, my family freaked out as I became visibly too thin, but I could not maintain this course. I got seriously hungry, and the pressure on me to eat what they ate was enormous. I eventually started to eat conventionally again, but my relationship with food remained problematic and unhealthy. I survived my teen years and managed to maintain a "normal" healthy weight despite my issues.

At age twenty-one, I got married for the first time. My husband's military assignment took us to South Dakota, which was far from friends, family, and everything I knew. There was no internet or cell phones. I felt very isolated and lonely.

I wanted to be a good wife, just like my mom. She made dinner for my dad every night, and I would do the same. I had my Betty Crocker and Time-Life cookbooks, and I knew how to follow a recipe. I also had learned quite a bit about making Italian food from my family. I was a fan of Julia Child and the Frugal Gourmet. It turns out I am an excellent cook, but at the time, I had zero idea how to make a meal nutritionally balanced. I was cranking out meatloaf, lasagna, and chicken pot pie daily. I gained about fifty pounds in the two years the marriage lasted. For various reasons, primarily due to my being unhappy and depressed, I was divorced at twenty-three. I moved back in with my parents and spent the next two years fighting to return to a healthy weight.

I was mostly healthy for a good stretch. I had been blessed with my Italian grandmother's smooth olive skin. I rarely sunburned, always tanned, and skated through puberty without pimples or acne. My brothers both needed glasses and had asthma, which I miraculously seemed to have escaped.

I would have happily never gone to a doctor, but my mother had now learned that DES had been known to cause a slew of problems, including but not limited to cancer, infertility, deformities, birth complications, and a host of other issues for both the mothers who took the drug and the babies who were exposed to it in the womb. As these babies of the fifties, the sixties, and early seventies grew up and more side effects were being discovered, I was pressured to have regular doctor appointments and screenings.

Fortunately, despite my exposure to DES, it seemed that my complications and side effects were minimal. However, if the studies have shown anything over the years, it's that they really don't know what the long-term effects are for DES victims or their descendants. I was found to have a somewhat deformed uterus, most certainly from the DES, and am considered high risk for cancer, but otherwise seemed to be doing ok, and was told to get screened yearly.

I felt healthy well into my twenties and went about my life

not thinking about my body other than my preoccupation with my weight, which predictably was now fully manifesting into an obsession.

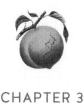

CHAPTER 3

I THOUGHT I WAS OKAY... UNTIL I WASN'T

Change is inevitable, and little did I know that what seemed like a straightforward decision to move in with my new boyfriend in Maine would have significant and lasting consequences that would irrevocably impact the rest of my life.

His house was heated by oil, and being one of those hardcore New Englanders determined to get through each winter on just one tank of oil as a matter of pride, he had this crazy idea that the hot air from the clothes dryer was "free heat." He intentionally vented it into the basement, saying, "The furnace wouldn't have to work so hard" if the basement was warmer, which would make the oil last longer. In addition, a drain in the cement floor backed up when it rained. Conditions were perfect for mold. After a rainstorm, that basement would look like the set of a sci-fi movie, and you knew that something creepy and scary was living down there. I would imagine monsters and swamp creatures hiding behind the stacks of boxes or junk, when in reality, the mold was the real danger, and it was *everywhere*. Not just a little mildew in the corners or underneath the washing machine, but Stephen King movie-level mold, with several inches of greenish fuzz growing on anything left down there for any length of time.

There was no telling my boyfriend what to do, so I sucked it up and looked the other way. I knew it was bad for us, but I didn't think it was worth fighting over. When I first moved into that house, I was never sick. Sure, there was the occasional cold or sore throat, but nothing noteworthy. I knew that mold wasn't good for you, but when you are a healthy twenty-something-year-old, you think you are bulletproof, and that "mumbo jumbo" about mold being harmful to you is all Bullshit.

When I say it's all Bullshit, I'm specifically referring to the attitude that was instilled in me by my dad. I remember he had stockpiled chemicals in his basement: insect sprays, cleaning products, and maybe some industrial lubricants. Stuff he was proud of because you couldn't find them anymore after the sale of them had been banned. As a child, I remember him explaining that he was lucky to have "the good stuff" and not to worry about why it had been banned because that was "all Bullshit." For the record, my dad is a fantastic person whom I adore. He meant no harm but was misguided when it came to certain things. I never saw my dad get sick, so he probably thought he was bulletproof. Maybe he is — currently, at 89 years old, he is going strong.

Headaches were the first of many mysterious symptoms, which, in the beginning, I could ignore, or at least power through. I had never had many headaches, but now I had them regularly, enough to be noticeable. Then, I just never felt well anymore. Nothing specific, nothing to see a doctor about. I just didn't have a lot of energy. I constantly felt like I was on the verge of the flu. I was tired much of the time.

While living in Maine, I worked at a factory. It wasn't exactly a dream job or a career path that I ever expected to be on. But on the other hand, I didn't know what I wanted to do with my life. I had already drifted through different jobs in my young adult life and had no real direction.

Initially, my job at the factory was to bond copper to beryllium ceramic chips by passing them through a screaming hot giant oven on a long conveyor belt. These parts would be used as circuits for hot/cold coolers and some for the space shuttle or the space station. We would load the pieces onto an automated machine that ran the oven and conveyor belts. The pieces needed to be perfectly lined up when the robotic arm deposited them onto the conveyor belt, or the circuit would be defective.

But sometimes, the chips would jam as they came out of the hopper. My job was to reach into the machine, pull out the jammed piece, and then jump out of the way before the robotic arms slammed back into place. As a safety mechanism, light bars were installed to trip the machine into shutting down if you leaned into the robotic arms' field of movement and crossed the light beam. But the engineers had disabled these so we *could* reach into the machine without stopping production, causing all of the product in the oven to be overcooked and ruined.

I knew this was wrong but I needed the job, so I did what I was told. One day, as I leaned way in to unjam the machine, the trapped ceramic chip shattered unexpectedly, and the robotic arms slammed into me, twisting my neck and shoulders with great force. I was injured enough that I was sent home to recover. After a day or two, I had improved, so I returned to work and did not give it much thought.

Eventually, I was moved into the screen-printing department, where liquid lead was screened onto beryllium chips for starter modules for GM vehicles. At first glance, everything seemed safe. It was a "clean room," and everyone wore lab coats, booties over their shoes, and hair nets. As I got to know my teammates, I learned that many of them had developed asthma and needed an inhaler. The reason for this became apparent fairly quickly.

Beryllium is an element used in manufacturing many electronic products because it has unique thermal conductivity properties. However, it is highly carcinogenic and considered to be toxic to humans at a similar level as arsenic or mercury. According to the National Institute of Health, it can cause berylliosis, dermatitis, acute pneumonitis, and chronic pulmonary disease and can be life-threatening from just small exposures.

My job was to feed beryllium chips about the size of a piece of Chiclet gum into one hopper, and pour liquid lead into another. The lead would be screen-printed onto the beryllium chip and run through an oven on a conveyor belt, which fused the two elements together. The "official" operation called for us to carefully examine each sealed plastic bag full of beryllium chips before we opened it. If we found even one chip that was cracked or broken, we were to return the whole bag to the supplier. Since beryllium was so toxic, the official procedure stated that we could not open a bag with a chipped or broken piece since there could be microparticles that could be released and potentially harm people.

In reality, though, we were always running short on our beryllium supply, and there were quotas to meet. So, every bag got dumped into the hoppers regardless of what it looked like, with an occasional bag provided to the engineers just to make it look like we were following procedure. Nearly all the bags had broken chips, which would have brought production to a standstill. I witnessed bags so full of shattered chips get dumped into the hopper that a cloud of dust would poof into the air.

I generally thought most of the precautions were "all bullshit." Even to me, this seemed potentially problematic, but I needed the job, and I was young, naïve, and *bulletproof*. I was also raised with my grandmother's stories of factory work and how she eventually became a well-respected supervisor at a shoe factory. I came from hardworking immigrants who instilled in me a certain work ethic; getting the job done was the most important thing. I didn't like my job but accepted that I didn't need to enjoy it. It was necessary, and that was that.

Weird stuff started to happen to me at work. Even before I moved into screen printing, I'd be out on the manufacturing floor, and suddenly, one of my eyelids would swell up. Out of nowhere, it would start to feel itchy, and then it would swell so fast I could see it happening when I went to the restroom and looked in the mirror. The first time, I assumed that a mosquito or a bug bit me on the eyelid while I was focused on the assembly line, and I didn't notice. I know how ridiculous that sounds, but I could not fathom what was happening. I was grasping for straws so I wouldn't have to go to a doctor. The swelling mostly went down by the next day, so I had nothing to show a doctor anyway.

A lot of the circuits we made were coated with gold. The gold needed to be salvaged if the circuit was scrapped for any reason. The room where they used cyanide to chemically strip the gold off the circuits was right next to my work area, and it always smelled horrible. On the one hand, I'd think, people work *in* that room every day, so it *had* to be safe. I started to wonder if maybe I was breathing too much cyanide, but then I decided I'd be fine when I got into screen printing. I'd be safe there.

That was the first time I considered a possible connection between the chemicals I was exposed to and my health. But ultimately, I decided that it was "all bullshit" – they couldn't have us working there if it wasn't safe, right?

When it happened a second time, again at work, I had to admit there were no incredibly clever mutant factory-dwelling mosquitoes that had a taste for my eyelids. So I left work and went straight to the emergency room while it was happening. The doctor there had zero idea what to do with it. He told me to put ice on it and go home. When it happened a third time, I saw a different doctor in the emergency room and was told I was having an allergic reaction to something unknown and to take Benadryl, put ice on it, and go home—nothing to worry about.

Then I started having neck and shoulder pain, and the mobility in my right arm started to be limited. The doctor I consulted examined me and found nothing wrong. He referred me to an orthopedic surgeon, who gave me a diagnosis of bone spurs and recommended surgery. I decided to get another opinion before committing to surgery and went to a second orthopedic surgeon. This doctor said nothing about bone spurs; instead diagnosed me with bursitis and also wanted to do surgery.

I couldn't understand why each surgeon gave me a different diagnosis. It made me very nervous, and so I opted to do nothing. I got a prescription for muscle relaxers and anti-inflammatories and went on my way. The internet was in its infancy, not as it is today, making it easy to look stuff up. At the time, if the doctor told you something, you either believed it or got a second opinion and then hoped the second opinion backed up the first opinion. Beyond that, there was the library and additional doctor exams and opinions.

I lived in that moldy house for five years and worked at the factory for the final two. When I first arrived in Maine, I was in my mid-twenties and never gave my health a second thought. Now, five years later, I was comparatively a physical wreck. I had headaches all of the time. My right arm and shoulder didn't work correctly anymore. I was always tired and a little queasy and constantly seemed to be fighting off a cold or flu. I became moody and depressed.

My boyfriend broke up with me. I don't blame him; I was not the same fun, healthy person who moved in with him, and in fact, was now miserable all the time. I didn't have the energy or the ambition to do much more than I absolutely had to. I did not enjoy being around me either at that point.

The break-up probably saved my life.

I moved out of his moldy house and eventually wound up back in Massachusetts and, at thirty-something years old, was living with my parents again. It was a little disheartening and not where I expected to be at that point in my life, but I was thankful that they were there for me. My parents had retired to Cape Cod and lived about a mile from the beach. I arrived at their house in late spring/early summer with visions of sleeping late, spending the summer relaxing, and going to the beach every day. I'd worked non-stop since I was a teenager, and I'd never had a vacation or time off. I was now in constant pain, didn't feel well anymore, and was ready for a break.

On my first night back with my parents, Dad proudly

informed me that he had lined up a landscaping job for me. I would be working for a local developer he knew, and I was to start first thing the following day. My parents looked at my shocked expression and said, "What? Did you think you were just going to lie around on the beach all summer?" I wanted to cry. I was grateful he had gone to the trouble of setting this up for me. I understood that I needed a job, but just once, I wanted to be that person who got to goof off and be a bum for a while. My parents didn't know how much I was struggling physically, mentally, and emotionally, and thought they were helping me.

I was not in the habit of sharing how I felt, so it's not their fault they had no clue how devastated I was. I was raised a certain way, so I sucked it up and went to work. The beach was still there for me on weekends. It was great being back with my parents. I was so tired on so many levels. I'd been through a divorce and then the breakup of a five-year live-in relationship, moved multiple times, and now had these health issues. I was still young but had been dragging myself through life for years, forcing myself to put one foot in front of the other.

Sometimes, you just want your mom to take care of you, and I so badly just needed her at that point. My parents and I had gone through a rough time in my teen years, and I had never really gotten to know them as an adult. I could now appreciate my parents in a way I never had as a child or a rebellious teenager. It turned out they were actually interesting, kind, and fun people. Even though they weren't about to let me be lazy for a whole summer, or at all for that matter, I still loved every minute of being back with them.

While living with them, I landed a decent job as a customer service rep in a call center for the local gas company. I was still plagued with neck and shoulder pain and headaches, and the mobility issues with my right arm would come and go. I now had excellent health insurance but no better luck with doctors than in Maine. I was not going to have surgery on something when I could not get more than one doctor to agree on a diagnosis. One of my bosses at work suggested that I see a chiropractor. I had no idea what a chiropractor was, much less had any thought about going to one, but he referred me to Dr. Dan, and I thought, what the hell, why not? This decision changed my life.

Dr. Dan did full body X-rays on me before our consultation. The doctors who wanted to perform surgery on me had each done precisely one X-ray, one on my neck and one on my shoulder. In the new X-rays, which were comprehensive and included entire body and spine images, Dr. Dan showed me - literally in black and white - that I had scoliosis. It had been missed when I was a child when it still could have been corrected. On top of that, the incident at the factory had aggravated it, causing additional injury, and none of it had ever been addressed. He proposed a non-invasive treatment plan that would get me to a good place, and then eventually only regular maintenance would be needed. I followed the plan and had my life back within six months. It felt like a miracle.

CHAPTER 4

BEGINNING, AGAIN

Things were going well. Living with my parents had soothed my soul. I'd recovered enough physically that I mainly felt "normal" again. Once again, I did not give much consideration to my health because, despite the physical struggles I had gone through for several years, I now thought of myself as generally healthy—mostly.

The eye swelling thing still happened from time to time, and I still had no idea what caused it. The headaches had eased up when I left the factory and moved from Maine, but never completely disappeared, which was frustrating and annoying, but not debilitating. The neck, shoulder, and arm pain issues were under control now through regular chiropractic treatment. I was generally okay. I moved on with my life.

I dated here and there, but never seriously. Then I took some night classes and met Dene at one of them. The teacher paired us up for some exercises, and we immediately hit it off. We started dating and eventually got married, bought a house with a yard, and adopted a dog. Life was good. After a couple of years, Dene talked me into starting a window treatment business with him.

It was far outside my comfort zone, but I knew how important it was to him, so I agreed.

We worked incredibly hard to build our business and became very successful. Initially we worked out of our home, but eventually we leased a small office with storage space. We added employees and company vehicles and our business grew, so we expanded to an actual showroom with offices and a warehouse. I devoted much time and resources to decorating our showroom and office space. We were in it for the long haul and were willing to lay the foundation for growth. We painted and renovated everything, installed new carpets, bought new fixtures and furniture, and spent a fortune on samples and displays.

We worked a lot. Even though we lived on Cape Cod, a resort destination, we had very little time off during the summer when the weather was good, because that was the busy season for our business. But still, we made time to go to the beach on some weekends and spent time with friends and family. My parents were nearby, so I got to see them regularly. I loved our house and had a flower garden that I obsessed over. I grew tomatoes in the summertime, always striving to replicate Grandpa's tomatoes. We had dogs that I adored. Life was good.

Our business was doing well. Dene was out in the field selling most of the time while I ran the showroom, answered the phones, and did the bookkeeping. For years, this had me in the office for very long days, often six days a week, eight to fourteen hours a day in the busy season. I was under a lot of pressure and stress all the time. Not only is it hard to start a business from scratch, but working as a husband and wife team is a challenge. We tried to keep our marriage and our business separate, but sometimes it got intense. Having children wasn't on our radar because the business took up so much of our time, and I wasn't sure I would be able to because of the DES.

The years slid by. I started to notice that I could always smell the carpet. It wasn't new anymore, but it began to seem as if the 'new carpet smell' got more assertive instead of fading away over time. Then, I became aware that when customers came into the showroom, I noticed what they smelled like, in a way I never had before. Specifically, if they were wearing some kind of fragrance, whether it be perfume, cologne, or just the laundry smell from their clothes, I would start to have an adverse physical reaction.

I found myself instinctively stepping back from people in an attempt to maintain my personal space and not breathe in their personal products and fragrances. Suddenly, I was physically struggling to distance myself from customers in the showroom. A shocking number of these people were utterly oblivious to this. When I stepped back, they would take a step forward, and I would find myself in an awkward little dance until I was crammed up against a wall, a display, or piece of furniture, dying for a breath of air, but too polite to tell them to back off!

Gradually, I started having new health issues that could not be explained. The headaches came back with a vengeance, and the eyelid swelling returned on a regular basis. I also started getting extremely painful boils on my butt or along my panty lines, making walking or sitting uncomfortable or sometimes unbearable. I had aches and pains all over my body.

My perfect vision now sometimes blurred, seemingly randomly, and my right eye would get goopy. I started avoiding driving at night because there were annoying halo effects around any lights, making it hard to see, especially in the rain. My eye doctor could find no cause for it.

I started having chest pain, heart arrhythmia, and palpitations. I didn't sleep normally anymore. I seemed to be breaking out or swelling somewhere on my body constantly. I didn't feel well most of the time and had started to gain weight.

Doctors didn't really have any answers for me other than advising that maybe I had food allergies or telling me I should try to lose weight – like I hadn't thought, actually obsessed, about that. It became clear the only tool in their toolbox was to throw drugs at me to manage a few symptoms, while the cause remained a mystery.

I went to an allergist/ENT, and his only option was to test me for the usual allergen suspects (pollens, animals, etc.) and then give me weekly allergy (SCIT) shots for the following indefinite number of years. He didn't know what was wrong with me, but he felt that if I got the shots, over time, it would help reduce the load on my immune system, and then some of the symptoms might lessen or go away. That seemed reasonable and made sense to me.

I started treatment right away and continued it for years. It did help with my fall hay fever, but the other symptoms continued to worsen. The doctors then told me it was likely food allergies causing my symptoms, but had been unable to identify which foods, and the shots didn't address food allergies. I tried to figure it out on my own by eliminating certain foods, but the results were never consistent.

I was about eighty pounds overweight. My weight had become an increasingly sensitive subject for me and not one that I was, or am, comfortable talking about. It has been a critical factor in my self-esteem and confidence — or lack thereof — my entire life. I am always painfully aware of my weight, even when it's in a "good" place.

During a visit to a new ENT to discuss my symptoms and lack of progress, even after years of treatment, he offhandedly commented that I'd be healthier if I lost weight. Then he said, "Maybe you should just not have that second helping of cake." I was stunned. Who the hell was he to look at me and conclude that I'm fat from eating too much *cake*? We had *just* discussed that I was struggling to figure out which foods I could or could not eat to try to manage my symptoms. (Cake was certainly not one of these foods.). How dare he say that to me?

I had been incredibly frustrated with my situation for so long, and here was this fool telling me to stop eating cake! I was highly offended. Everything in me wanted to scream, "Fuck you! You fucking fuck!" But I was not a confident enough person to defend myself. So I did nothing. I still gave doctors automatic respect and authority, even when they had not earned it. The person I am today would have a *very* different reaction.

This was not the first nor last doctor who would look at me and declare, "You should lose weight," a statement I found profoundly unhelpful. Did they honestly think I was unaware of this fact? I was never offered any help or solutions, so they were just giving me shit, fat-shaming me, and giving me one more thing to feel frustrated and helpless about while I was already at a personal low.

Over the years, my frustration with doctors grew, and my respect for them dwindled. My aunt told me she had gone to a local acupuncturist to treat her shoulder pain and mentioned that the acupuncturist also offered treatment for food allergies.

I was ready to try a new route. Maybe *this* would save me. I thought food allergies were at the root of most of my problems, so I made an appointment.

I had never been to an acupuncturist before and knew nothing about it other than they stick needles into you. It was not something I was looking forward to, but I was willing to overlook that if it would help. The process starts with the acupuncturist taking your "pulses." She put her fingers over my wrist and "listened" to my pulse along different sections of my artery. She looked at my tongue and asked me some questions. Then she told me, "You're really toxic; your problem isn't food allergies, it's toxins, you are full of them, and we need to treat your liver and detox you."

What? This was completely unexpected, and I didn't want to hear it. I had gone there to get treatment for food allergies, not to sign up for a lifetime of acupuncture trying to detox my liver. What the hell was she talking about? Wasn't she listening to me? Couldn't she just stick some needles into me and I'd be done?

She did a treatment that day, which wasn't the painful experience I was expecting. Tiny little hair-thin needles mostly in my feet, hands, and face, really no big deal - I barely noticed them. But I didn't feel any different afterward, and she told me I needed to commit to a regular and reasonably aggressive schedule for a long time if I wanted results. I felt like it was a trap or a trick. My health insurance didn't cover acupuncture, and I just saw an endless future of me throwing money away on this. I decided not to go back.

New symptoms continued to appear. The flawless skin I'd had all my life was now often broken out in a rash or rosacea on my cheeks. I developed adult acne. My doctor was starting to question if I had Lupus but decided first to send me to a dermatologist. When I mentioned the chronic eye swelling problem to the dermatologist, he casually said, "Oh, that's angioedema; you're probably sensitive to salicylates, which are found in certain foods." He gave me a list of foods high in salicylates, told me to avoid them, and sent me on my way.

I was stunned, shocked, speechless. How many doctors had I told about the eye thing, and that was it—this guy nails it in two minutes? It was hard to believe, but I was thrilled to have a diagnosis and *specific* actions to take. All I needed to do was avoid foods high in salicylates. No problem, easy-peasy. I was very good at having an unhealthy relationship with food; I could make this work and get back to normal. I embraced that list as if my life depended on it, which I believed it did. *Finally*, I had a plan.

Except it didn't work. Not exactly. Sometimes it did, and sometimes it didn't. I quickly identified oranges and tomatoes as two of the worst offenders, so along with a slew of other fruits and vegetables, I focused on eliminating anything with salicylates from my diet. Suddenly, the foods I had eaten all my life were off-limits, but that would be fine if I got my life back, right? So much for the search for Grandpa's perfect tomato, I had bigger problems. I made lasagna with cream sauce instead of tomato sauce. I drank cranberry juice instead of orange juice. I'd look for pizza with white sauce. This was a solvable problem.

Salicylates are found in most plants, and ironically, the plants that are higher in salicylates are also typically healthy foods that lower inflammation. I didn't know yet that my inflammation was extremely high, so I severely limited fruits and vegetables, opting for more meat, fish, dairy, and eggs. This new diet seemed to work ok for weeks, and then suddenly, I'd have all kinds of symptoms, and I wouldn't be able to pinpoint what I had eaten to set it off. I'd been so careful! It was incredibly frustrating.

By this time, I had to hire someone to help me at work because I no longer had the stamina for the long hours, and the headaches made everything harder. Sometimes I'd be sitting at my desk, and I'd feel like my lungs were burning, my skin was itching, and my head hurt so bad I couldn't see straight, but I had a job to do, so I had to suck it up. I was not sleeping well, and the boils were irritated by my clothing. They weren't only painful, but also embarrassing. I felt ashamed. It seemed like it was somehow my *fault* that this was happening. Because I couldn't explain it, I thought it looked like I had done something wrong. I hid it for years.

No one except my husband, Dene, knew how miserable and uncomfortable I was nearly all the time, or that I was so often in terrible pain for no apparent reason. I was living a secret life. I was incredibly relieved that at least these things were not on my face or where people could see them, but it meant no one knew what I was going through.

No one knew how miserable I was, and consequently, couldn't understand why I didn't want to do anything. Even something as simple as going for a walk was painful for me most of the time now. I struggled to get through each day. And my now unbalanced and unhealthy low-salicylate diet caused more weight gain, which made me even more miserable. My doctor had no answers. I was desperate for relief.

Someone told my husband about Anthony William, the Medical Medium, a famous self-proclaimed medium who offers pseudoscientific health advice based on alleged communication with a spirit. Although he no longer does appointments for readings, at the time, you could enter a lottery for an appointment. On a whim, Dene entered my name, and after about six months, I was contacted and told Medical Medium would do a reading for me. On the one hand, I had never heard of this guy and thought it seemed pretty out there. On the other hand, I was ready to try anything and figured there was no harm in it.

During our phone consultation, he told me I had Epstein Bar Virus and that my body was full of toxins. He said the virus was entrenched in my organs and would not show up in a blood test. He gave me a list of things I needed to do that would help me over time. Hold on, was this guy in league with the acupuncturist telling me I was full of toxins? His instructions included going completely vegan, eating only organic whole foods, and he gave me a lengthy list of supplements to take. I was most definitely not prepared for that.

Gone was the little girl who did not want to eat meat, especially now that I had been leaning heavily on meats because I avoided salicylates (more commonly known as *fruits and vegetables*). I had been expertly cooking steaks and barbecuing ribs for years now. I was excellent at using dry rubs instead of BBQ sauce since tomatoes were "Public Enemy Number One." I owned four grills and two smokers. I wasn't cut out to be a *vegan*. I'd cooked a pig on the beach! If I cut meat, fish, dairy and eggs out of my diet, *and* still avoided salicylates, there'd be nothing left for me to eat. For several months, I half-heartedly took some of the supplements he recommended. I tried and failed to adjust my diet and eventually forgot about the whole thing.

I bumbled along, trying different combinations of food avoidance. I continued to operate on the premise that salicylates were causing everything, even though the results of my carefully constructed diet experiment no longer supported that theory. I still desperately clung to it like a drowning woman because I needed *something* to blame. Things continued to get worse.

I had started taking sleeping pills. They worked for a couple of years, but eventually not so much. I continued to take them anyway, fearing I wouldn't have had any sleep at all. But now, I was sleeping only a couple of hours. I would have trouble falling asleep, and then I'd wake up after just half an hour with pain in my whole body. I'd roll over, fall back asleep eventually, and then, in another thirty minutes, wake up in pain and start all over again. On average, I was getting a grand total of less than two to four hours of interrupted sleep at night.

A strange side effect of the sleeping pills was that I began 'sleep-eating,' or whatever you want to call it. I'd lie awake in bed, waiting for the pill to take effect, sometimes for hours. The longer I stayed awake, the more I became fixated on how hungry I felt, frustrated that the pill hadn't worked yet. Eventually, I'd give in, get up, and prepare the most bizarre food combinations. I didn't realize at the time that I was already somewhat impaired by the drug. Eating seemed to trigger the pill's effects, and finally, I'd get sleepy, go back to bed, and sleep soundly for a few hours. This did not help with my weight problem.

More symptoms gradually crept in, each more troubling than the last. I constantly felt the urge to urinate, even when my bladder was empty. I had mysterious unexplained pain throughout my whole body. Major brain fog set in, making it impossible to remember things unless I wrote them down. I struggled to express my thoughts clearly, as the right words seemed to slip away from me. The headaches intensified, becoming so severe that I could barely function, with no relief for weeks on end. Nausea became a constant companion, often leaving me feeling disoriented and unable to see straight.

When you live with this intensity of constant headaches, it's hard to describe what it's like to go through the day-to-day process of living your life. I had a business to run—I had to go to work. It didn't matter how much pain or discomfort I was in. I still had family obligations and always a to-do list. There was no point complaining; that just made people uncomfortable. It wasn't like they could do anything to help me.

It took all of my willpower to get out of bed each morning. I had no energy to do anything that was not mission-critical. I had painful boils all the time now. I felt very, very alone. This was sucking the life out of me —invisibly. No one knew the level of hell that I was going through except for Dene.

I no longer thought of myself as a healthy person.

I was now forty-five years old and had not felt well in years. I liked my general physician/PCP, whom I had seen for many years. She was great when I'd get a sore throat or was due for a pap smear, but all of this other chronic stuff was beyond her expertise.

When I got new health insurance, I had to choose a new doctor in my new HMO network. I was hopeful this new doctor might know something. I eagerly set an appointment. Maybe *she* would be the one to help me. I was so optimistic when I told her everything I had been experiencing. She looked at me and said, "Well, you have an irritated bladder. I'll write you a prescription for that. I'll also provide something for you to try for the headaches, though I can't guarantee how effective it will be. Your miscellaneous pain is probably caused by fibromyalgia or polymyalgia. I'll prescribe prednisone for that. You'll probably have to take that for the rest of your life. I don't know what's causing your angioedema.; Keep working on your food sensitivities. I'll give you muscle relaxants for the pain and more sleeping pills. You might have Lyme disease, but that's hard to nail down. I can refer you to a rheumatologist if you think you want to go to one."

I was shocked. Why did I ever expect her to be any different? By now you'd think I would have learned not to get my hopes up. I went home to my husband, five new prescriptions in hand, and broke down in tears.

"I don't understand. I'm only forty-five years old. I feel like an old lady. This doctor just gave me prescriptions for someone decades older than me with serious diseases. I don't think she has any idea what's wrong with me either. I think I'm going to die soon. What is happening to me?"

At that moment, I was giving up. I had no hope for my future and was ready to die. In fact I welcomed it.

CHAPTER 5

AN ACTUAL DIAGNOSIS

Dene listened to everything, looked at the prescriptions the new doctor had given me, and said, "We'll find your answers. I'll help you." He truly believed there was an answer and that the power of the internet could help.

I had lost my faith in doctors and had no hope for my future. You could now add depression to my list of problems. It sucked the life from me just as much as the constant pain and discomfort I was in. I threw away the fistful of prescriptions, well, except for the sleeping pills and muscle relaxants. I was depending on those. I never went back to that doctor.

Dene's research turned up "Dr. L," an environmental doctor who was relatively nearby, only a couple of hours' travel time away. After reviewing the information on her website, we realized that I was very possibly "environmentally ill" and contacted her office for an appointment. Her assistant sent me a *twenty-seven-page questionnaire.* The questionnaire was simultaneously a shock and gave me hope again. This doctor was actually asking questions like: "Have you ever been exposed to mold?" or "Have you ever been exposed to heavy metals or toxic chemicals?"

ARE YOU KIDDING ME? Why was this the *first* time anyone had thought to ask me these questions? In a flash, it all seemed so obvious! Oh My God! Years of living in that moldy house and then working in the factory being exposed to all of those toxic chemicals - suddenly it was as if I was struck by lightning! Even as I was filling out the questionnaire, I *knew* this was the problem. Every single other doctor had seen me as a collection of symptoms and threw prescriptions at me to treat them, never trying to understand why or what was causing these symptoms in the first place. But this time, I just knew it was going to be different. It was like a weight was lifted from me before I met with the doctor. I was about to reclaim my life. I couldn't wait to meet with her.

I completed and sent in the questionnaire and scheduled an appointment as quickly as possible. In the first of what was to become commonplace for me in this next phase of my chronic illness, my insurance did not cover this; she was out of network. I went to see her anyway. She set up an array of tests. Anything that came out of my body was collected, shipped out, and tested, and I mean anything and literally everything. I was spitting in tubes, pooping in cups, giving hair samples, and collecting my urine in a giant jug. I provided so many blood samples that I wondered if there was a daily limit on how much they could take.

The results? I was environmentally ill and chemically sensitive, sometimes also called Multiple Chemical Sensitivity or MCS. That was good news - wasn't it? I had an actual diagnosis now. I wasn't crazy. The bad news was that it's not exactly curable. There are treatments, sort of, so the disease can be managed, sort of, but there was no magic pill that was going to cure me.

In addition, it's not mainstream medicine and is still generally considered experimental by insurance companies, so almost none of my treatments would be covered. It would all be time-consuming, uncomfortable, painful, inconvenient at best, and always expensive. The prognosis was indeterminate, in part because it was not yet clear how much of the recommended treatment I could afford or take time off work for. Even if I had unlimited funds and time for treatment, results could still be unpredictable for this kind of affliction. Then there needed to be more testing, sometimes stuff I had never heard of. But this was a start. It was something to grab onto, more than I'd had in years.

I did the "tilt table" test at Mass General Hospital, which was bizarre. They strapped me flat to a table, put in an IV, attached a multitude of electrodes, and put a blood pressure cuff on one arm. Then they tilted the table to about twenty or thirty degrees and took readings. Nothing happened. The doctors running the test commented to me that doctors typically find this test very boring to perform because usually nothing happens. Then, they tilted the table again to about sixty degrees.

All hell broke loose. Suddenly, the blood started draining out of my head super-fast. I could literally *hear* it happening. It sounded like one of those rain sticks that make noise when you flip it around, and all the seeds inside drop to the bottom. I was instantly nauseous and felt like I was about to shit myself and faint. Not good. I could hear the doctors in the room shouting at each other. One yelled that she was trying to get a reading but couldn't. It sounded like they were in a tunnel and getting further away by the second. I heard them saying they couldn't find my pulse or blood pressure. They kept asking me to talk to them and to hang on, but I could feel myself blacking out.

When they lowered the table back to flat, I instantly felt the blood rush back into my head, reverse rain-stick style. They let me lay there for a while until we all felt like I was stabilized. I asked them what was in the IV that did that to me, and they said nothing – the IV was just saline, and it was there in case they needed to inject something quickly. My reaction to being tilted was purely mechanical. The whole thing was crazy. I had fainted more than a few times in my life but had never realized it could be induced literally by simply *tilting* me. I've thought about this a lot since, wondering why I haven't been fainting all over the place if that's all it takes. But actually, there are never any occasions where my body is straight, which is apparently a critical component, and also simultaneously tilted at a specific level.

I met back up with my new environmental doctor and got an additional diagnosis. The tilt table test confirmed Dysautonomia, sometimes referred to as POTS disease, which is a fancy way of saying that I am fainter. More importantly, it means my Autonomic Nervous System is impaired. That's what controls or regulates our bodily functions automatically, including heart rate, digestion, blood pressure, etc., so it's kind of important. POTS disease is not curable, but it can be managed and seemingly was more of a secondary problem. Millions of people have dysautonomia, many of them unaware of it, and live without any real inconvenience.

I had multiple brain MRIs, and they found lesions, likely due to a severe fall when I fainted in a 99 restaurant while I was still living with my parents on Cape Cod. I remember waking up on the floor, surrounded by strangers, to the words, "At least someone should pull her dress down over her panties for God's sake." That's something you never want to hear. I was mortified beyond belief. My head was exploding, and I was having trouble focusing my vision, but my only thought at that moment was, "Why are people looking at my underwear?" Someone kept telling me to be calm; the ambulance was coming. I felt someone else pull my dress down to cover me up. (Thank you, whoever you are). I was so embarrassed the first thing I could think to say was, "I'm not drunk!" Because I wasn't, I'd had a few sips of a beer and a few bites of food. I struggled to get up and asked for the check so I could exit this nightmare. I immediately fainted *again* and hit the floor *again*.

I woke up in the hospital, where they ran tests, pronounced me concussed, and sent me home. Later that week my PCP would tell me that I likely had low blood sugar after not eating all day. Years later, the dysautonomia diagnosis would make me re-examine this event because clearly, my Autonomic Nervous System had been malfunctioning for years and was likely a significant player in that event.

I now had a lot to learn. I thought I had a pretty good idea of how I got there, but did I? Was it all just the moldy house and the factory? I learned there are so many factors in environmental medicine that it's almost impossible to pinpoint one cause. I had fainted multiple times in my life going back to my teen years, so the Dysautonomia had been going on for decades, perhaps my whole life.

Did the chemical sensitivity then really start in Maine? Or did it begin before I was even born when my mom took DES and laid in bed drinking wine and smoking cigarettes all day — following doctor's orders? Did I miss out on something important because I was fed meat goop instead of breast milk? I was a smoker from age 14 to about 41; all those years of smoking certainly didn't help my situation.

I learned that we all have a "bucket" that handles the toxins we put into our bodies. Mostly, the liver is the "bucket," but not entirely. A healthy "normal" body filters toxins through the liver, and then hopefully, all or most of them are processed and flushed out, generally at a rate that keeps the toxins from accumulating too much or too fast. Some, like mercury or other heavy metals, are stored more permanently in the liver, brain, fat cells, and elsewhere. When a person overfills their bucket or puts a particular combination of toxins into the bucket, it can be like a switch turning on/off, and suddenly, they are "flipped," sometimes called "tilted," and they become environmentally ill and chemically sensitive.

Once that switch is flipped, *everything* changes. Suddenly, every chemical in your environment, on your food, in the air you breathe, in the personal products you put on your skin, what you wash your clothes in, all go into your bucket. Your liver no longer has the ability to process these toxins out of your body fast enough, and your bucket is always full. Symptoms begin to appear.

Everyone's symptoms are different and unique because each person's body is different and unique. The combination of environmental exposures that cause their switch to flip, along with the new triggers that set off their symptoms, is unique as well. This complexity is part of what makes diagnosing environmental illness so incredibly challenging.

As I have come to understand and to put it in simple terms, environmental medicine and chemical sensitivity are all about emptying the bucket, detoxifying, and identifying and avoiding additional toxins or exposures. This would now become the focus of my existence: emptying the bucket and avoiding new exposures.

At first, this seemed straightforward. After all, I no longer worked in a factory or lived in a moldy house. How hard could it be? If I thought avoiding oranges and tomatoes was annoying, I was in for a whole new level of inconvenience. My world was about to turn upside-down. I learned one of the reasons the high-salicylate-food-elimination-roulette-game I had played had such erratic results was because, at the time, I had no clue that it was not just the food I was eating that caused my symptoms but *also the air I was breathing and the products that I was touching or putting on my body!*

I did get tested for salicylate sensitivity at some point in my environmental medicine journey and was found to be level three out of five salicylate sensitive by the Mayo Clinic. So the dermatologist was not wrong; he just saw a small piece of the puzzle, a very small piece. Eating salicylates was only a problem if I ate too much of them *and* was exposed to other toxins. But at least now I understood why the results of my salicylate-restricted diet were so inconsistent – it wasn't just the salicylates affecting me!

I now needed to identify the toxins in my environment and remove them, all of them. How hard could that be? HAH! Remember the "new" carpet at the office that wasn't new anymore but still *smelled* like new carpet to me? I could barely tolerate being there anymore because of it, and had to move the bookkeeping part of my job to a spare bedroom at home. We hired someone to work in our showroom, greet customers, take deliveries, and answer the phones. I had become too sick to manage this part of our business alone. Although I still needed to spend time there for many of my duties, I also required significant time off for my treatment. It was a four-hour round trip for me to go to my environmental doctor, plus time there being hooked up to an IV, and I needed to do it multiple times a week.

I went on a rampage to rid my environment of toxins. The first thing to go was the carpet in the back offices at work. I was not sorry to see it go. This was commercial carpeting, and it was glued down onto a plywood base over the cement floor. When my staff tried to pull it up, it was like taffy or gum on your shoe; the glue had never wholly dried, and years after installation, it was still gooey and sticky and smelled like chemicals. It hadn't just been the carpet that I had been smelling and getting sick from. For all those years, I was in that windowless back office, often for more than twelve hours a day, breathing that glue, the carpet, and the plywood, all of which were off-gassing formaldehyde and who knows what other toxic chemicals. No wonder my bucket was full!

The doctor had many recommendations for me, all of them expensive, most of them inconvenient, and collectively, utterly overwhelming. I had to pick and choose what to tackle first. The easy part was personal and household products. By "easy," I mean not overly expensive or inconvenient compared to home and office renovations. Still, it's more complicated than you think to suddenly change every product in your life to fragrance-free when you have never really thought about it. Fragrances are in nearly everything.

Overall, we did a good job making everything fragrance-free right away. I had been eliminating products one at a time for years, thinking, "Oh, the smell of that gives me a headache." But I never realized just how many products were fragranced, or how they could be affecting me, even when I didn't think they were. Now, I made a conscious effort to target everything in my environment, which was a huge undertaking.

If you think I'm exaggerating, just read the labels on your products and see how many of them have fragrance listed as an ingredient. Check your shampoo, conditioner, hand lotions, shaving creams, moisturizers, deodorants, sunblock, hair gels, and hair sprays. Actually, sunblock, hair sprays, and gels, even when fragrance-free, are big offenders and generally not okay for chemically sensitive people. Remember, fragrance is the easy target, but it's the chemicals in fragrances, and the chemicals in everything else that I had become overly sensitive to. So even when something was labeled fragrance-free, that didn't necessarily mean it wouldn't affect me.

It's not just personal products either. Look in your kitchen at dish soaps, hand soaps, and dishwasher detergent. What are you cleaning your house with? If you have a cleaning person, they are almost definitely defaulting to using all fragranced products. Cleaning products are so tricky because they are nearly always fragranced on top of whatever their base cleaning chemicals are, which are typically problematic.

Then there's makeup. Many makeup products have a masking fragrance; it's very tough to find good fragrance-free makeup, lipstick, foundation, etc. It might not sound like a big deal to change out all of those products until you start shopping for fragrance-free or non-chemical replacements. Then, it becomes painfully apparent how fragrance has wormed its way into so many of our products. And again, it's not just the fragrance. It's petroleum products, stabilizers, pesticides, additives, plastics, heavy metals, and more.

I recently watched a limited documentary series on Max called "Not So Pretty." I highly recommend it to anyone interested in learning about what's in our beauty products. I was shocked at some of the information, and I've been reading product labels for years. For example, I had no idea that some of my make-up might have asbestos in it because apparently, *it's impossible to remove asbestos from talc, therefore all talc has asbestos in it!* I'm looking at you, baby powder and eyeshadow! It's like an upside-down world onion – you think you are seeing the whole picture, but every time you peel back a layer, there's another level of fuckery.

Am I being overly dramatic in using the word "fuckery" to describe what goes into our personal products? No. Because fuckery implies that somewhere up the line, someone or some group knows there are toxins in our products, and not only do they not care, but perhaps go to great lengths to cover this information up. Products that we trust and never in a million years would have suspected of having toxins, can make us sick. Do I sound paranoid? You don't need to take my word for it. Just google J&J ovarian cancer lawsuit, or watch "Not So Pretty" and then decide for yourself.

Next on the chopping block was our home carpet, which was extensive. Not only could I smell the formaldehyde wafting out of it, but carpets trap all kinds of toxins and allergens in their fibers. It had to go.

Ceramic tile is the recommended flooring for chemically sensitive people. We had natural wood floors on most of the first floor, which was fine because they had off-gassed years ago. I hated the idea of putting tile in the upstairs bedrooms, but I had gotten so overexposed to carpet at work that I had no tolerance anymore. We chose a tile that looks like wood planks. It looked *great* when it was done and was super easy to keep clean. This was a win-win if you don't count the expense and inconvenience.

We bought an organic mattress. When sleeping, our bodies are trying to repair damage, and breathing in toxins from a typical mattress was not helping. We found a fantastic organic mattress company, and Dene and I both slept better on the new mattress from the very first night.

Next up: my teeth. I had always taken good care of my teeth and was over thirty before I got my first filling. By forty-five, I had several. Unfortunately, they were traditional metal fillings, recommended by my dentists as the safe and affordable option that would last the longest. Dr. L was adamant they had to go; keeping them was not an option, as they were likely leaking mercury into my body.

From the FDA's website: "*Dental amalgam fillings may release small amounts of mercury in the form of a vapor (gas), depending on the number and age of existing fillings, and actions such as tooth grinding and gum chewing.*" And, according to the World Health Organization: "*Dental amalgam is used in almost all countries. A 2009 WHO expert consultation concluded that a global near-term ban on amalgam would be problematic for public health and the dental health sector, but a phase down should be pursued by promoting disease prevention and alternatives to amalgam; research and development of cost-effective alternatives; education of dental professionals and the raising of public awareness.*"

No amount of mercury is considered safe. How is it possible that I have had multiple dentists install this in my mouth as if it were?

This was going to be expensive. I have always had a lot of anxiety about dentists, so I was not in any hurry to put myself through an extensive procedure. When I did finally bite the bullet (so to speak) and got rid of the metal fillings, there was a noticeable improvement in my symptoms very quickly afterward. Side note: It's essential to work with a dentist who is familiar with this procedure and knows how to take great care to prevent any mercury or toxins from being released into your body *during* the process.

Food. I had never been in the habit of choosing organic, nor given it much thought. Now, I was *very* aware that every bite of food was potentially filling up my bucket of toxins due to the pesticides and growing practices of conventional farming. I needed to be vigilant about this. It's a good thing I already knew how to obsess over food.

My cookware? Yes, I had some stainless steel and cast-iron pans because I love cookware and kitchen gadgets, but my go-to was non-stick pans all day. It's the only type of frying pan I remember my mom ever having, and it's what I learned how to cook on as well. I had a history of years of misusing them, using high heat and utensils that scratched the coating, forcing a replacement on a regular basis. I'd heard they were bad for you but, again, thought it was no big deal; that's all bullshit. But now I knew these pans were *also* contributing to filling my bucket, so they had to go. I also threw away all the Tupperware and anything else plastic that stores food storage containers; plastic can leach into food.

And while we were in the kitchen, my natural gas stove had to be replaced with an electric model. I fought this one. I was one of those people who firmly believed you needed to cook with gas to get the best or chef-level results. There had been a gas stove in almost every kitchen of every house I'd lived in my whole life, how could this be part of the problem? Once I started paying attention however, I realized that whenever I was cooking on my gas stove or using the oven, my face and especially my nose would turn screaming bright red and get itchy. This had been happening for so many years I didn't even think about it anymore, and when I did, I blamed the food.

Dr. L kept pushing me on the stove, and like the tile floors, this turned out better than expected. I purchased an induction stove, which unexpectedly, I *loved*. Induction heats up faster than gas, is easy to clean, cools down fast when you remove the pot, and is safe because it will shut off if there is no pot on it. I've become a huge fan. And guess what? Gas stoves may be on their way out. Laws are being passed in some areas prohibiting gas appliances from being installed in new homes. This is a highly contentious and controversial subject at city, state, and federal levels. I expect it will continue to be a battleground for years to come, but I'm a convert and now much prefer induction.

I was incredibly annoyed to be told to make some of these changes with products I had thought safe my entire life, only to discover that my environmental doctor was right, time and again. Annoyed is an understatement; I was pissed off about so many of her instructions. I had to be pushed to make many of the recommended changes. In addition to all of the expense and inconvenience, I was *sick* and had trouble getting out of bed in the morning. Dr. L might as well have asked me to climb Mount Everest.

I am eternally grateful she had the patience to keep after me to make these changes despite my extreme resistance to many of them. Each of them seemed insignificant, but collectively they had been ruining my life. She was right.

I now had a diagnosis and a plan. This was something I could work with. I had an actual *villain* – toxic chemicals – that I could target as part of my new understanding of what had happened to me, and I had a plan to work my way out of it. I knew I had a hard road ahead, but I was hopeful and determined. I didn't have to climb that mountain in one day. I could chip away at it in my own time, some of it in baby steps, and other parts in giant leaps, but eventually I would get there.

CHAPTER 6

TREATMENT

I was excited to have a path to wellness, but at the same time, there was just so much; it was overwhelming financially, physically, mentally, and emotionally. I was taught from an early age to expect a certain flow to the world of medicine. If you are not feeling well, you go to the doctor; you trust that doctor; you get a diagnosis; the doctor prescribes treatment, and then hopefully you are cured, or you are given an accepted and well-known protocol to manage your illness. Generally, you expect your doctors to know what's wrong, explain it to you, and prescribe treatment. If you are lucky enough to have health insurance, you expect your insurance company to pay for most things. If your prognosis is grim, you can expect support, concern, and empathy from friends and family, or even complete strangers.

I was now living in a world where I finally had a diagnosis, but it was not widely accepted as a real thing - not by my regular PCP, not by my insurance company, and now I was discovering, not by some of my friends and family. My treatment plan was complicated, expensive, and a mystery to most people. I had to figure out how to prioritize my way through it based on what I could manage at any given time.

I changed my health insurance company, so at least the visits to my new environmental doctor were covered as in-network, but not much more. They covered the occasional blood test and her office visits now, but I had to pay for most other tests and treatments out of pocket. Still, I was committed to doing as much as I possibly could. I sorted my treatment plan into bite-size chunks and tackled the problem one piece at a time.

I managed the fragrance-free thing first, and an interesting thing happened. It's technically called "unmasking." When you stop inundating yourself with fragrance, your olfactory fatigue (which most people have) disappears, and you can start to smell things for real. I was already a good part of the way there, but now that I was militant about it, the resulting reveal was shocking. It was suddenly apparent to me that *everyone* was covered in fragrances and chemicals everywhere I went.

It didn't happen overnight, but between the unmasking and my new understanding of what had been making me sick, my perspective changed, and I was now hypersensitive on multiple levels. There was almost nowhere I could go that I was not suffering from some sort of fragrance or chemical. My home was now my bubble, my safe place. It became painful for me to go out, to leave the safety of my bubble, and allow myself to be exposed to the toxic soup that was the rest of the world. I still needed to go into our office and showroom, so I now needed our employees to be fragrance-free. Our staff was amazing. They were incredibly supportive and went to great lengths to accommodate me. I will always be grateful to them.

Dr. L had advised a staggering number of supplements for

me to take, along with several prescriptions. Although I despise pill-taking, I was all in. I wanted to be a good patient and do everything she told me within my financial abilities. I gagged those pills down every day—my new insurance paid for some of the prescriptions, but none of the supplements.

At her direction, we purchased a sauna and installed it in our basement. One of the side effects of my affliction was that I did not sweat normally and could no longer self-regulate my body temperature easily or appropriately. I'd get into the sauna and would not sweat for an uncomfortable length of time. Instead, I'd just be overheated and miserable at first. I would have to lie down in it and keep my head down so I didn't faint. Dene loved the sauna and always felt great when he used it, but I had to force myself to do it for a very long time. I found it uncomfortable and unpleasant. It was an essential part of my treatment, so I powered through it, and eventually, I would start to sweat when I went in.

I was going to the environmental doctor's office for regular IV treatments multiple times a week. The office visit was covered by insurance, but the IV treatments were not. From my door to her office, I traveled about two hours each way—not unmanageable, but not awesome either, especially if you don't feel well. I always felt worse *after* my treatment and was miserable on the ride home every time. I also still had a business to run and work at, so the regular treatment schedule was difficult, expensive, and inconvenient. I wanted to get well and was committed to my program.

I got worse before I got better. I learned this was what happens when your body starts to release toxins. Now, the toxins were no longer just sitting in my liver or fat cells but were now raging around my whole body and brain, looking for a new home. I still had all the same symptoms that I started with and even picked up a few more now that I was detoxing.

Dr. L told me there was another environmental doctor in Texas I needed to go to for a specific treatment only he could provide. She said he had invented a treatment that was an antigen made from the patient's own T-lymphocytes that they inject themself with on a regular schedule. She was chemically sensitive and had gone to him for treatment when she discovered she was environmentally ill, and it had been life-changing for her. She felt that, without that treatment, I was not going to be able to improve much more, and she strongly encouraged me to go to him for this. It would be another thing that she would push me on continuously until I eventually agreed.

None of the treatment in Texas was covered by insurance, but it seemed like the only path forward for complete healing, so I went. This was no easy decision, and not just because of the expense. Travel had become out of the question for me. I was now completely unable to tolerate any fragrances or chemicals for any length of time. An airplane flight would be torture, and then where was I to stay?

I was directed to a condo complex in Texas that rents to chemically sensitive people. This was a godsend. The condos had tile floors and furniture that didn't off-gas, and they didn't clean the units with toxic chemicals or wash the linens in anything fragranced. It was such a relief to stay there, and I will always be grateful to Earl, the owner, for providing a safe place for people like me.

I wore a mask on the plane, which is amusing now that Covid has made masks commonplace everywhere. At the time, I stood out like a pariah, being the only one on the plane or in the airport wearing one. It made people very uncomfortable. I never felt that masks did a great job of filtering out fragrance, so I was always on the fence about using them. I knew other patients who wore gas masks on planes, but that was beyond what I was willing to do, and anyway, those smelled like plastic and rubber to me.

At the clinic in Texas, I was immediately plunged into a comprehensive testing and treatment plan. I was subjected to a new slew of tests, including a brain SPECT scan, balance testing, thermography, and antigen testing. Days of nothing but antigen testing and getting poked with needles to test my sensitivity to a variety of potential offenders.

The list of antigens they could test for was extensive and included things you would never imagine. Like stainless steel, for example. Would you believe I am mid-level reactive to stainless steel? Of course, you could test endlessly for foods, pollens, animals, molds, and obvious things. But they could also test you for the not-so-obvious, like your reactivity to your own brain's neurotransmitters, like serotonin and histamine, just to name a few. They could test your reactiveness to perfumes, colognes, laundry, and cleaning products, or pretty much anything you could think of.

Most of the antigen testing was done in rooms where a group of patients sat lined up in front of the lab assistant, who would rotate through the patients, sticking each of us with needles and measuring the results every 15 minutes. We would all be in the same room together for this process, all day, every day. It was monotonous. I learned that when they move you out of that room for a different needle test that is not one of those usual antigens —prepare for it to hurt like hell. It's like when

TSA doesn't like the look of something about you or your bags, so they pull you out of the airport security line and bring you to a little room. You know you are not there because they're going to offer you a margarita.

The testing results allowed them to create antigen formulas for me to inject myself with regularly to lower my sensitivity to these items, along with the Autogenous Lymphocytic Vaccine, which was the main reason I was there, and the reason I received the extra painful needle testing in the little room. From my time in Texas, I would now have a new additional treatment: inject myself with these formulas every three days for years to come, or indefinitely. Initially, I would inject myself in the abdomen twelve times every three days. The needles were tiny, just little diabetic needles, so they were not really painful. But when you are doing twelve of them at a time, on the regular, it's not awesome.

They also set me up for Immunoglobulin Therapy for my PCP doctor to do at home. Since I was now used to injecting myself with needles all of the time, I couldn't understand why I couldn't just do this one too. They explained that this one was different. It needed to be injected into my butt and monitored by a doctor in case there was a problem or unexpected reaction. I wasn't nervous until the doctor brought out the largest needle I'd ever seen. As I was bracing myself for this thing, the doctor *literally* said, "Oh wait, I need a bigger needle; this injection uses the biggest needle I have." She actually left me in the room with that thought and this giant needle on the tray, and then came back in with another needle that was so big it looked like a movie prop to me. This thing belonged in a cartoon, and it was about to be jammed into my butt cheek! Not fun, nope, that was definitely not awesome.

I met a lot of other patients at the Texas clinic and got to know some of them reasonably well. After all, we spent many hours together in the testing rooms, where cell phones and books (paper and ink are triggering for many people) were not allowed. I spent a lot of time quietly chatting with my fellow patients and learned quickly that, as sick as I thought I was and had been, I was one of the lucky ones. I was fortunate to have found my way to an environmental doctor before becoming completely debilitated. If I thought I was miserable and my life was all about pain and discomfort, many of these other patients that I was getting to know were in much worse shape.

Many of them had started out chemically sensitive, and without treatment, progressed into electrical or EMF sensitivity. Discovering this shook me to my core. I had developed a fairly low-level sensitivity to EMF by then, but it was manageable. Mostly, I would find that I couldn't tolerate long conversations on the phone without breaking out into hives, so I always used speaker phones and never put my phone near my head.

These people were experiencing an entirely different level of misery. They could not go anywhere where they would be bombarded by Wi-Fi or cell phone waves or other electronics (which is almost everywhere these days), or it would result in potentially excruciating reactions and symptoms. For them, it was similar to what I experienced from perfume or laundry products, and for some of them, it was at a life-threatening level. Many of them couldn't use a phone or a computer at all, and this was *in addition* to avoiding chemicals and fragrances.

I had found avoiding chemicals and fragrances to be hard; I could not imagine having *also* to avoid electronics and Wi-Fi. Some of them could not ride in cars without being affected, and flying was out of the question. One woman I met could hear bits of telephone conversations of people talking on cell phones, even just driving down the street and talking on the phone in their car while she was on the sidewalk. I met patients there who could not tolerate most food, or were triggered from fabrics in clothing other than unbleached organic cotton. I learned that some patients become homeless because they cannot tolerate building materials anymore, and some of them even lived in tents in their backyards because of this.

Now that I understood that things could be so much worse for me than what I had already been experiencing, I was more determined than ever to be a good patient and follow the treatment plan. I spent years being fragrance-free and avoiding toxins and exposures, doing regular saunas, taking supplements and prescriptions, getting IV treatments, and injecting myself. I went back to Texas about once a year and got retested to update all of my antigens and formulas, and I continued to inject myself.

I had four tattoos that I had gotten as a teenager and in my twenties. It was determined that the ink in at least one of them had mercury in it. So, I spent years having them lasered off. It was expensive, painful, and inconvenient. My first several treatments were a nightmare. You can smell your skin cooking during the lasering, and it hurts more than getting the tattoo in the first place. For me, especially the first five or six treatments, it was equivalent to at least second-degree burns, sometimes worse. The first few times, the tattoo on my left leg turned into a blister the size of a baseball and got infected at one point. I had to wait for the blisters to turn into scabs and then for the scabs to go away before my subsequent treatment, so my early treatments were at least a couple of months apart. It took a couple of years to laser my tattoos off, and I have scars now from the lasering.

When you break up a tattoo with a laser, the ink has to go somewhere, right? You don't want it to just decide on its own to take up residence in one of your organs with all that mercury and who knows what else. So, I made sure to have corresponding IV treatments and injections of glutathione right after lasering and throughout the process. Glutathione injections are expensive, inconvenient, and not fun, but they are one of the only ways to get mercury out of your body. Of course, none of this was covered by insurance.

I'll never forget the day Dr. L told me that test results indicated I needed to give up gluten, dairy, and eggs. Gluten was first. I was in the office with her for one of my regular appointments, and she told me new test results indicated that gluten was a problem for me, and it had to go. I thought about it briefly and said, "OK, I can do that; it's not like you're asking me to give up cheese."

Gluten-free was manageable. It was a little tricky, but I could do it. After all, I was an old pro at obsessing over food. Over the next couple of weeks, we transitioned into a gluten-free household. I became an expert at converting recipes. I even started to relax about it and thought, "This isn't so bad."

On my next appointment, the doctor told me, "You need to give up dairy also." That one just about brought me to my knees. I *love* dairy products. I love milk and cheese and ice cream. Wright's Dairy Farm in Rhode Island was about an hour's drive from our house, and we used to get fresh milk and other dairy products there. I had never had farm fresh milk before I had milk from Wright's Dairy Farm. Until I went there for the first time, every glass of milk I had ever drank in my entire life came from a grocery store shelf. I was shocked at the difference and really had been enjoying the good stuff now that we had discovered it.

Wright's also has an insanely good bakery, which I had already resigned myself to saying goodbye to because of the gluten, but now the milk too? Oh my god, that was a knife in my heart, but again, I sucked it up and did what I was told.

When I first got my diagnosis, I was so focused on my treatment that I was not careful about what I was eating other than trying to keep it organic to avoid chemicals and pesticides in my food. In addition, I didn't feel well most of the time, so I did not have an exercise routine. For a long time, I was just trying to survive. Consequently, I gained weight, but because I had so many other issues, I forgave myself. I would live with it or figure it out someday in the future, but for the moment, I did not have the bandwidth to tackle that particular problem along with my other treatment. My food options were becoming more limited again, and I needed to figure that out first without worrying about being on a "diet," too.

Before giving up gluten, I had been experiencing increased heart palpitations and chest pain for a while. These symptoms had become a daily occurrence, and so Dr. L referred me to a cardiologist. He did a full workup, including sending me home with a heart monitor for a weekend. It was right after that weekend that Dr. L had me give up gluten. Then, it was another several weeks before I had my follow-up appointment with the cardiologist to review the results of the stress test and heart monitor.

The results showed I was having heart arrhythmia multiple times a day. As he started to advise a drug-based treatment plan for me, I told him that within several days of giving up gluten, all of my heart symptoms went away. By the time I was sitting in his office with him that day, I had not experienced any chest pain or palpitations for some weeks! He looked at me and said, "You know, that's so odd. You are the second patient this year who is telling me something like this."

I chose not to take any medications for my "heart condition" and instead just committed to being gluten-free. The heart symptoms did not come back as long as I was gluten-free. I have experimented with this over the years and learned that I can have some gluten occasionally, but if I get too cavalier about it and eat it more than occasionally, then the symptoms come back.

I came so close to being put on statins when all I needed to do was eliminate gluten from my diet. How many people take heart meds when they only need to adjust their diet? And why didn't this cardiologist know that could be a thing? Clearly, I'm not the only one with this type of sensitivity. I'm not suggesting that everyone stop taking their statins or heart meds and try going gluten-free all of a sudden. I am saying, however, that I was learning the hard way that I needed to have a voice in my treatment plan.

I continued to get better. Not cured, and not "normal," but better, improved. My symptoms slowly eased over the years. Initially, it was like having the flu or a virus all the time. In the beginning, if I had an exposure to something triggering, it would affect me for weeks, or sometimes longer if it was particularly bad. I would refer to this as having an "exposure hangover." After more than five years of treatment, I knocked that down to about a day or two. This was a big deal, and I was extremely pleased.

Remember the acupuncturist who, way back in the beginning, told me I was toxic? I returned to her and said, "You were right; I'm full of toxins!" I started regular acupuncture treatments with her, which I found to be highly beneficial. Little by little, I was reclaiming my life.

Eventually, I realized I had plateaued in my treatment. I was working in my office again and could live "normally" in some ways, but some things were still entirely out of reach. Travel was still not manageable for me other than in the RV we had purchased because of my limitations. I was better on an airplane than before, but most hotels were still out of the question. Laundry products remained the bane of my existence.

I became frustrated that my treatment was not bringing me the total freedom that I craved and had *expected* to have by then. It had been years; why wasn't I living a totally normal life? How long could I keep up this plan's financial, emotional, physical, and mental strain? How long would the people I loved put up with it? It wasn't just a hardship for me; it was a lot to expect from my friends and family. They were constantly being ticketed by the fragrance police, *aka me,* and endlessly being asked to bend over backward for things that they couldn't understand, smell, or sense.

I was sick to death of the pills, the needles, and the expense; I came to a point where I didn't want to do it anymore. It was also frustrating that I could not effectively determine which part or parts of my treatment brought me the most relief. Was it one or two things, or was it everything? I needed to take control.

It's hard when you constantly shell out money for prescriptions, and the insurance company won't reimburse you for anything because they consider it all "experimental." You start to question what is real and what might be a placebo. Their refusal to accept my condition and my treatment was not just a financial burden, it also eroded my confidence in the entire treatment plan. After all, insurance companies paid for many expensive surgeries, treatments, drugs, and hospital stays for everybody else – or at least that's what it felt like. Why was my illness and my treatment not covered? Wasn't I worthy? Was I not sick enough? Was my illness not real? Did they think it was all in my head? It was beyond unfair, and it really affected me mentally as the years went by.

I now suspect that insurance companies take this position for multiple reasons. First, because it's so difficult to diagnose, it's slippery enough for them to blame the diagnosis as not real so they can get out of paying. But more significant than that, if they recognize the problem and environmental medicine becomes more mainstream, and more people with chronic unexplained symptoms are diagnosed with environmental illnesses, the cost of suddenly treating potentially a *substantial portion of the population* would be financially devastating.

Remember how the World Health Organization recognized that just targeting metal fillings in teeth would be a financial disaster? Imagine expanding that beyond the dental world to include all of our environmental exposures. I suspect the potential number of people with undiagnosed environmental illnesses is significant enough that suddenly covering the expense of treating even a *fraction* of them would be catastrophic to an insurance company.

I was tired of it all and started to wonder if there was another path.

CHAPTER 7

LIVING WITH CHRONIC ILLNESS AND CHEMICAL SENSITIVITY

If your illness is of the "hard-for-other-people-to-see -evidence-of" variety, you learn quickly that you are on your own when you leave your house. Patients with clear and obvious physical afflictions get plenty of sympathy and consideration comparatively.

Chemically sensitive people and persons with other invisible or unfamiliar diseases generally do not receive the same consideration as persons with prominent or well-known afflictions. In fact, the opposite is often true. We can be treated with disrespect, annoyance, and even outright disbelief. Sometimes, people assume we are mentally ill and that we should be able just to get it together and move on.

For a chemically sensitive person to leave their house and interact with the world is an act of courage every time. Grocery stores, restaurants, town halls, train stations, airports, hair salons, government buildings, arenas, churches, hospitals, doctor's offices, schools, malls, and public spaces, just to name a few, are minefields that require precise planning and strategy.

I had to get a doctor's note to get out of jury duty because I could not possibly sit with the other jurors and not be affected. I would be constantly distracted by all the potential smells and exposures in the courtroom. Not only could I get sick, but it could also affect my ability to think clearly and be an impartial juror.

Going to a restaurant – assuming you are well enough to go into one at all and can find food on the menu to eat – could look something like this:

We tend to go to restaurants during the slowest times to mitigate the number of people we are exposed to. Then, we carefully assess the seating and try to manipulate the situation so that we are always seated with the most space between us and other people. If we are in a group of friends or with family, I can promise that they are all in varying degrees of "safe" to be near or sit next to, so we strategize where to sit for optimal results between the people we are with, and potential strangers around us.

Once this maneuver is successfully executed, we secretly wait in terror to see what the server smells like or anyone seated near us. If someone covered in laundry or perfume is seated at a table nearby after you have ordered your meal or drinks, what do you do? Do you ask to be moved? Do you ask for them to be moved since they have not been served anything yet? But then, if you ask for them to be moved, are you expecting the restaurant not to put anyone there now? Can you even ask the restaurant to try not to seat anyone overly fragrant near you? I have actually done that more than once with varying results, most of them not positive.

What about the waitstaff? If they are covered in perfume or laundry or both, every single time they come over to the table with a drink, or food, or to refill your water or pick up a dish, it's as if they punch you in the face. Think about it. In most of these instances, they pass their arm right before your face, in front of your nose. So if they have any fragrance on them, you will be on the receiving end of it. Repeatedly.

What do you do? Do you ask for a fragrance-free server? I have done that on more than a few occasions when my self-preservation instinct would override my need to be polite and my fear of making a scene in a public place. I've long since gotten over being worried about offending someone by making these kinds of requests, but that doesn't mean anyone with me feels the same way. Sometimes, it is accepted with grace and taken in stride, but not always. So, do you just suck it up and spend the rest of your meal in survival mode? Or do you get up and leave?

Bravery takes many forms for a chemically sensitive person. What if you need to use the restroom? Is one of those fragrance machines installed near the ceiling? God help me when I see one of those. It's bad enough when I'm desperately trying to navigate all the restaurant employees and other patrons, and possibly cleaning products, but those "air fresheners" are their own particular category of hell. Not only do I need to hold my breath and get in and out of there as fast as possible, but if it happens to shoot a blast of its chemicals while I am in there, now it is on me and in my hair, and I can't get away from it.

What about the soap in the restroom? Assuming there is some, it doesn't matter; I can't use it anyway because it's almost always fragranced. Not only that, but I can't let the other people in my group use it either. If someone else goes to the restroom, washes their hands, and then comes back and sits next to me or is going to get in the car with me, then we are playing fragrance roulette. If you will be in the car with me, you can *never* use the soap in any public restroom. I happily will supply you with a travel-size squeeze bottle or a medical wipe from a pack I carry with me, but *please* don't use their soap and sit next to me or get in my car.

Why am I making such a big deal of this? Why don't I just shut the fuck up and deal with it so everyone can have a nice dinner?

When I am being exposed to someone else's secondhand fragrance the best way to describe it is that I feel like I am eating it. I can literally taste it. If I'm in a restaurant and my server is wearing something, especially scented laundry products, I become overwhelmed with the smell and taste of it, and it eclipses everything else, including whatever I am drinking and eating. It sucks up all of my sensory input bandwidth and leaves me with no room for anything or anyone else.

It is so all-encompassing I can't redirect my brain to focus on anything else, and I am reduced to obsessing over how I will escape it. The last thing I want to do is eat anything at that point. If my companion is talking to me, I am incapable of properly attending to the conversation. I become unable to process anything other than the feeling of toxic chemicals assaulting me directly through the blood-brain barrier. I instantly start to have impaired functioning and cognitive ability. Depending on the exposure, various symptoms begin to present themselves quietly and invisibly. It's torture.

It takes a massive amount of courage for the average chemically sensitive person to attend a public event or gathering, go to a wedding or graduation, eat in a restaurant, or shop in a store, and we do so in general for the benefit and consideration of those that we love and care about. Symptoms can be anything from mild headaches to stroke and everything and anything in between. There is a lady's perfume that, when I am exposed to it, causes me to develop painful sores inside my mouth within five minutes. It's invisible to everyone else but very real and painful to me.

Occasionally, I might say to someone who is a close-talker: "Excuse me, I'm allergic to certain perfumes and fragrances; forgive me if I need to step back a bit." You would think I had slapped them in the face, that suddenly *they* were the victim of *my* incredible thoughtlessness and rudeness, as opposed to the physical suffering that I was already beginning to endure and could potentially expect to endure for days to come due to my forced exposure to their secondhand fragrance. Am I ranting? Yes! Your *perceived* right to wear whatever you want is infringing on my *actual* right to breathe clean air.

I have also found that my sensitivity to a specific product often escalates the more I am exposed to it. So if someone in my circle starts using a particular product that I initially thought I could tolerate, the more I am exposed to it, the less I am able to tolerate it. It's very frustrating to both of us when something they thought was on my approved list suddenly becomes a problem, and I start complaining about it.

Another particularly offensive product is fragranced deodorant. When I am near someone wearing fragranced deodorant, and it is wafting around, I feel like I am licking their armpits.

When you are chemically sensitive, you don't smell fragrances the way the chemists design them to be experienced. It's more like you are "tasting" not just the fragrance parts of the product but also the underlying chemicals that go along, like the stabilizers, preservatives, solvents, and carriers - chemicals that make the fragrance waft around and *stick* to things. Oftentimes, it's similar to biting down on tin foil if you have metal fillings. It's a sensory overload in a fingernails-on-a-chalkboard way.

Certainly you can *never* use hand sanitizer around me. That stuff can be horrific, and it's everywhere since Covid. One time, I was at the hospital being checked in for a brain MRI, and the intake person, without warning, squirted a giant glob of a well-known hand sanitizer onto the counter and her hands just as I sat down. It sent me into a fit of sneezing and snotting that would not let up. When I got loaded into the MRI machine shortly after, they put a cage on my head to immobilize it. I had stopped sneezing but was still super sniffly, and my nose was still running. I lay there in the MRI for over 30 minutes with nasal discharge pooling in my ears and behind my head because one person liberally applied a common scented sanitizer right in front of me moments before the test. How could she have known? I don't expect her to have, but I would expect the hospital to know better and adequately train their personnel in fragrance-free protocol and policy.

Doctors' offices, hospitals, and testing facilities seem to be full of people who smell like the stinkiest laundry. Whenever I was scheduled for any testing, I dreaded it as I always felt like the other patients smelled like laundry, personal products, and fragrances more than anywhere else. I mentioned this to Dr. L once, and she responded that it was not my imagination; she said the people in these waiting rooms had a much higher percentage of being fragranced than the average population because people who use fragranced products get sick exponentially more than people who don't, partly because their immune systems are always overloaded.

What about cars? Buying or renting a car, riding in other people's cars. Cleaning and maintenance of vehicles. Letting other people ride in your car? All very complex problems requiring an enormous amount of planning, strategy, and research.

Simple everyday activities, like grocery shopping, can be daunting. Many chemically sensitive people can't go into a grocery store at all. They sell soap and shampoo, laundry, and cleaning products there, so of course, that's a problem. The people in the store with their various scents are problematic. I hate it when they put the paper towels too close to the laundry products because it contaminates the paper towels right through the plastic.

Since we mostly eat fresh fruits and vegetables now, I rarely spend much time in the middle of the store, which is helpful because that's where most of the smelly stuff is. I hate it when fragranced people get close to the organic vegetables though, because when the misters come on, the fragrance molecules get trapped in the mist spray and then are misted onto what *was* an organic product but is now contaminated. I also hate it when store employees contaminate the products by touching things if they have fragrances, lotion, or sanitizer on their hands.

I am mystified when I smell a person loaded with fragrance and see them buying organic produce. Don't they know they are so covered in chemicals that those organic apples will never offset all the damage they do to themselves with their laundry choice? Sometimes, their toxic chemicals affect my brain enough to disengage my filter, and I will approach them and tell them what I am thinking. Without exception, this has never ended well. Do I believe that one day, one of these people will look back at me and say, "Thank you, I had no idea. I'll definitely make better choices moving forward, and I'm sorry that I assaulted you today." What's wrong with me? I know that will never happen, yet I do it anyway.

Movie theaters, shows, theme parks, fairs, casinos, and concerts are all off the table. Any place where I must be seated next to strangers is a no-go. Casinos have the advantage of allowing you to keep moving if you are playing the slot machines, so if I am lucky enough to find one that is non-smoking, I go when it is not busy, like 6:00 a.m., before they clean the carpets, then I'll have a fighting chance of having a good time. Of course if you are in a Las Vegas casino, they pump fragrances in through the ventilation systems now, and there is no escape from that.

At some point, while I was still pretty sick but had improved enough to take some chances, Dene and I decided to take our parents to Las Vegas. My parents had never been, and I was determined to "suck it up" so we could have this experience together. I did a lot of research and booked "stay well rooms" at the MGM Grand. They use non-toxic cleaning products and have special air filters in these rooms, so I thought it would be okay. The rooms turned out to be manageable for me. Unfortunately, we had to walk through two miles of vanilla-scented casino to get to the room.

The MGM signature vanilla scent was sickening and pervasive. You could not escape it. Even in my fragrance-free stay-well room, I could smell the chemical vanilla scent coming off my clothes and hair from walking through the casino. We all had dinner at Wolfgang Puck's Bar and Grill one night; all I could taste was that horrible vanilla fragrance. Every bite of food was tainted with fake vanilla, and I felt like I was eating a bar of soap.

I actually went to the trouble of hunting down a hotel manager. In retrospect, I realize my filter had disengaged because of the exposure. Otherwise, I would have realized this was pointless. I explained to him that we were paying extra for the stay-well rooms, but we had to go through the rest of the casino to get there, so everything got contaminated anyway. I also explained that the vanilla scent had made the dining experience very unpleasant.

This guy then proceeded to mansplain to me that *all* the hotels now had a signature fragrance and that it was necessary to "manage" the cigarette smoke. I looked at him and said, "But you know the cigarette smoke is still there, right? You know we're not fooled by this vanilla fragrance; we all know we are still breathing secondhand smoke; we're not stupid."

Needless to say, the letter of complaint I sent upon arriving home received no reply.

I was not able to go to a mall at all for years. Eventually, I was able to do surgical strikes and targeted quick shops. Now, I can go longer without problems, but I still find it challenging to purchase clothes at stores that sell fragrances. Anything displayed for more than a day or two begins to absorb the fragrances from the store. The length of time an item is exposed seems to correlate directly to my ability to de-stink it when I get it home. This is a struggle for me even now, because so many of these chemicals won't just wash out of the clothes.

Before I became sick, I always assumed the clothes I bought

in a store or online were "new." It is rather shocking how often I have purchased something, and then when I have it at home – and away from the store's fragrance counter – I can smell laundry products on it. This means someone wore it enough to feel obligated to *wash* it before returning it, or they wore it long enough for the laundry smell to ooze out of their pores and infiltrate the fabric. I can also tell when it's been dry-cleaned and returned.

If someone else purchased an item, washed it in fragranced laundry, and returned it, it's ruined forever. If it's been laundered, I always return it because there's no way I can de-stink it. If it's perfume, either by contamination from the store or from someone who tried the item on, then I will usually give it a shot with my multi-step decontamination process. This involves sandwiching my new clothes in multiple EnviroKlenz Odor Eliminating Pads, stuffing it all in a bin, and leaving it for days or weeks. Eventually, this will eliminate many fragrances but not laundry. There have been times when I bought something new, and it was a solid year before I could de-stink it enough to wear it. At that point, it may not fit anymore, or quite simply, I'm just not that into it anymore. There have been times when I have washed a new garment so many times to de-stink it that it would start to pill, shrink, or otherwise be ruined before I wore it even once.

Chemically sensitive people have to think about what furniture they are buying. Is it going to off-gas? We have to think about everything we bring into our homes – appliances, paint, flooring. We need to consider electronics and wi-fi as most of us are also EMF-sensitive. Landscaping must be carefully thought out because we can't tolerate chemicals for weeds or non-organic fertilizers. I once had thirty yards of mulch delivered, only to realize I did not receive the organic mulch that I thought I ordered, and consequently, I couldn't spend time in my yard or open a window for weeks. Also, we can't just willy-nilly spray for insects or termites without careful research, consideration, and planning.

What about pets? Cats must have fragrance-free litter in their boxes. Dogs may need to go to the groomer, so their shampoo needs to be fragrance-free. And you might need to supply your own towels for the groomer to use on them. You need to pick your dog up the minute the grooming is complete so they don't get covered in secondhand fragrance from the shampoo the groomer uses on everyone else's dog.

We obsess about who is coming into our house. It was ironic that I got too sick to clean my own house, but then I could not find a fragrance-free cleaning person to do it either. Whenever we need a plumber or an electrician it seems like they are always doused in the smelliest of laundry products. Here at our new house, we've had the Geek Squad from Best Buy come out to install some electronics. I tell those guys every time they come that they are killing me and themselves with their personal products. I can see their eyes glaze over while I am talking to them. Nobody seems to care, and I know I look like a crazy person to them.

Where people like me choose to live presents another set of hurdles. First, there cannot be any hint of mold or mildew in our living space, house, or apartment. Next, what about the local outdoor air quality? Places with a lot of smog, such as Los Angeles or Salt Lake City, are bad choices. Places that do a lot of fracking and oil drilling, like parts of Texas, for instance, are also terrible choices.

Apartment or house? Rent or own? What is the neighborhood like? Are the lots small and the houses close together? If the neighbors use scented laundry products, I won't be able to be outside when they do laundry, so the more neighbors there are, the more I won't be able to be outside. My house is my safe place, my bubble. The very thought of moving into an unknown environment is terrifying.

What about work? I was fortunate that Dene and I owned our own company, which allowed us to control the environment. It's bad enough that when you are sick all of the time, you don't feel well enough to go to work. But to have your workplace make you feel even worse is just soul-crushing. Most of us need to work and have no choice, so we suck it up and force ourselves to deal with it.

Being chemically sensitive has made me realize there are also things we should be thinking about for our pets. It is a scientific, undisputed fact that dogs have an extraordinary sense of smell. According to the American Kennel Club, a dog's sense of smell is estimated to be as much as one hundred thousand times more sensitive than humans. I can't even wrap my brain around this number.

Dog brains are also different from humans, designed to process smells with such complexity that we can't even imagine what their experience is like. Research has shown that using their sense of smell, dogs can detect cancer, low blood sugar, diseases, viruses, and migraines, to name just a few. Dogs have even been known to predict seizures before they occur. According to *understandinganimalresearch.org*, in a 2006 study, dogs could detect breast cancer with 88% accuracy and lung cancer with 99% accuracy across all four stages of these diseases.

I can smell laundry products on a person across a busy parking lot without even trying, and I'm just a human. What is it like for my dogs to be subjected to that level of secondhand fragrance? What is it like for a dog to be bombarded with all the smells, perfumes, and fragrances in an average person's house? What is it like for them to lie on a carpet that has been "deodorized" with a fragranced product or have their hard-surface floors cleaned with scented products, their nose right on top of that stuff? What is it like for them to go to the groomer and come back immersed in scented products? If it pains me with my enhanced sensitivity, which is truly only a *fraction* of their olfactory abilities, what is it like for them?

What is life like for other people with sensitivities or allergies?

I can only speak to my personal experiences. I know that it's different for everyone. There are plenty of things I have no clue about, and another chronically ill person reading this might be annoyed, wondering why I left out obvious things that make their life miserable. But that's the thing with environmental illness; it's different for everyone.

Living this way is incredibly difficult, complex, and over-whelming. Much of the time, our issues are invisible. We are all too aware of how annoying and inconvenient our particular needs are to the people around us. We constantly straddle the line between self-defense and trying to power through so we don't alienate the people we love and care about. Even those closest to us have no idea what goes through our heads when we receive just a simple request to meet a friend for lunch. We are not looking for attention. We just want to be normal.

CHAPTER 8

TRAVEL

It is difficult to fully describe what it feels like not to have the freedom to travel like a normal person. It's completely demoralizing and frustrating on so many levels. It seems like everyone I know is constantly posting about exotic places, fun trips, cruises, and special events, and I have to strategize just to go to a restaurant.

In chapter one, I painted a picture of what it's like for me to attempt to book a trip and then what happens when I actually try to go through with it. Sometimes, we'd wait years to go on a vacation. We would save our money, and I'd be so careful planning it, or so I thought, yet more than once, it would turn into a disaster. I'd wonder, was I really going to have to tell Dene that I couldn't stay in the room that I so carefully vetted and booked, but it made me sick when we got there? What was I to do with that? If he wanted to divorce me, I wouldn't blame him. It all felt like insanity to *me*!

One of the difficulties of being chronically ill is how it affects your family and everybody around you. I was marginally okay with being a prisoner of my disease, but it wasn't fair for Dene to be a prisoner, too. I've been incredibly fortunate with how Dene has handled all of this. I was committed to figuring out how we could enjoy a more normal life - together.

So what do you do if you just can't travel like a normal person and need to find alternative solutions? If you can't afford to fly private or own multiple homes, then what? You realize that an RV is the answer! You can bring your safe bubble with you everywhere you go. Of course, you know you'll never be able to go anywhere overseas in your RV, just North America, but so what? You will still get to take vacations and travel, right?

For starters, what kind of RV are you going to buy? You can't just rent one for the same reason that you can't just rent any old car or stay in just any hotel room. So, how do you go about buying an RV?

It's even more difficult and complex than buying a car. If it's a used RV and the previous owner used a formaldehyde septic tank additive (before that stuff got banned), then that smell is going to infiltrate everything in your camper, so that's a no-go. Or if the previous owner used scented laundry products, you know by now that you'll never get that smell out.

Therefore, you'll probably have to buy a new RV. What's your budget? They can be somewhat affordable for a smaller tow trailer, or you can spend millions for a rockstar-style bus. However, affordable ones are not a viable option. They are designed to be very lightweight so they can be pulled by SUVs or even cars. The downside is that the materials they use to make them can be very toxic. These trailers are not intended for people to live in them long term; they are designed for people to stay in them for short vacations, so high amounts of formaldehyde and other toxic glues and chemicals are considered acceptable for their construction.

There are very sobering stories about what happened to the people whom FEMA housed in inexpensive trailers after Hurricane Katrina. If you pop into a new one of these affordable, lightweight trailers to check it out, the chemical smell is so overpowering it's like a punch in the face. Even people who are not sensitive can smell it. They are not an option.

What about a motorhome? Generally pricier than a lot of the travel trailers, but not quite as bad, right? Yes, but...they still have a lot of particleboard and glue in them and, consequently, a lot of chemicals off-gassing. Motor homes start to fall into the category of the more you spend, the more likely you will be able to get one that is not off-gassing like crazy. But how much do you have to pay?

Good question. I have spent an enormous amount of time smelling new motor homes with prices ranging from $70,000 to $600,000, and they *all* off-gassed chemicals to a noticeable degree. Some of them have some carpet, or it comes from the walls, the furniture, and the cabinets. Would it all off-gas and eventually be okay? Sure, some will, but there's no telling how long that will take. Do you have someplace indoors to store the motorhome with the windows open while you let it off-gas? And that's another thing too: where will you keep your RV?

If you have millions to spend, then you can get something custom-made that won't have those issues. At least I assume so, as I have never had that kind of budget any more than I have the budget to fly private, so I have not investigated that option. But it makes sense that if you have millions of dollars to spend on a custom motorhome, you can have it custom-built with materials that won't off-gas and affect you. For the rest of us, however, we are relegated to choosing from the off-the-rack options.

After I got sick and we realized I could not travel normally anymore, we bought a used 2001 Coachmen Class C motorhome and renovated it to make it as non-toxic as possible. It was extraordinarily difficult to de-stink it, as the previous owners had used products that contaminated it. For many years, however, it was still a much more viable solution than a hotel or Airbnb, enabling us to take vacations and travel.

Our current camper is an Airstream travel trailer. This camper has metal walls and ceilings, so it has far less material in it to off-gas. Even so, we let it sit in our driveway for about a year before we started using it, and I still run an air filter in it most of the time when we stay in it. We replaced the original mattresses with organic, and I typically use an electric hot plate instead of the propane stovetop. I was able to live in this camper full-time for many months quite successfully after we sold everything and moved out of our house in Massachusetts.

Is it the perfect solution? Not by a long shot. We had to buy a new truck to pull it, for one thing, and although I could drive the last camper by myself without a problem, pulling a travel trailer is a different kind of driving and not one that I am well suited for. Dene doesn't mind it though, so he does all the driving when we go somewhere with it.

Camping can mean a lot of things, but most of the time, it's not like the pictures in brochures or the television commercials that show happy families frolicking by a picturesque sapphire blue lake with Bambi posing on the edge of the campsite and no one else in sight, just miles of gorgeous forest and majestic mountains in the background. It's usually very different from that.

We have camped everywhere, from full-service beachside resorts to "dry camping" or "boondocking" out in the wilderness to parking in a friend's driveway and everything in between. RV parks range from basic and roadside to luxurious and waterfront, sometimes spectacular, sometimes a little scary. We have been fortunate to stay in some truly amazing locations and have had many unforgettable experiences. There are a lot of benefits to traveling this way, but also there are plenty of compromises.

Camping is not the perfect answer, but it is *an* answer, and it has been a way for us not to be imprisoned in our home. When camping, I'm usually able to limit the amount of time I spend around people or in places that have too much chemical exposure for me. I always pack a massive amount of clothes into our camper since it has no washer/dryer. I can't use the washers/dryers at the campgrounds because they are contaminated with scented laundry products. I can cook in it, and it has a decent-sized fridge/freezer, so we don't always have to eat out when traveling.

Another benefit of traveling by RV is that, in general, our dogs always get to come with us on a trip. It's difficult for us to leave them behind for any reason, not the least, because they are like children to us. Why wouldn't we want them to accompany us on a vacation? Traditional travel methods and lodging are problematic if you want to bring your pets. Traveling by RV usually solves that, and I love that about camping. Our dogs are our family, and we are all happiest when we are together.

There was a time when I started to think I would never be able to leave my house again. It's a deeply sad and lonely feeling. I began to develop a mindset that I was just waiting to die. I felt like I had no future. I like to think that I have reclaimed some of my freedom, at least enough to feel "kind of normal," and I have camping to thank for much of that. We've had some fantastic experiences camping, and of course, some unpleasant ones too. I consider myself very fortunate to be able to travel this way – with Dene and our dogs.

Does this mean I will never get on a plane? No, I will if I have an overwhelmingly important reason. But I still generally avoid flying, and then, if I must go, I certainly do not look forward to it. Over the years, I have learned to set myself up for success by being strategic about the process.

I dream about a future when I can visit other countries or just travel without jumping through hoops or thinking about every possible detail. I watch friends and family plan trips without having to give any thought to what the linens might be washed in at their destination or what the rental car will smell like, and I am envious. But then I realize I have so much to be thankful for, and I let it go.

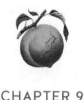

CHAPTER 9

RELATIONSHIPS

I t's difficult to express what my life is like to someone who is not sensitive to chemicals and fragrances and, therefore, has no context from which to relate. This book is my attempt to do so.

As I already pointed out, I don't just smell chemicals and fragrances; I *taste* them. Fragrances and chemicals affect every aspect of my life. The effect on my relationships was, and still is, monumental. The people in my life, especially my husband Dene, my friends, and my family, who have stood by me and bent over backward to accommodate me, are the true heroes of this story. These people have spent years adjusting their lives for me. Their personal product choices, which should have been private decisions, have been dictated by me, despite the fact that most of the time, their experience with these products is entirely different than mine, and they rarely smell things the way I do. Yet they have allowed me to influence their choices repeatedly without complaint.

Sometimes, people who truly care about me and are trying to be thoughtful are still very unaware of how their use of fragrance still affects me, even when we are not in person. They make an effort to be fragrance-free around me, but otherwise use it regularly. They don't understand that everything they own gets saturated with it, and even when they think they are fragrance-free, they are carrying their own second-hand fragrance with them into my house, my car, and my presence at a painful level. If you put cologne or perfume on for "special occasions," then I promise you it is now on everything else in your closet; it's on your furniture and in your car too. You just can't smell it anymore because you are in olfactory overload, and it's almost invisible to you.

Unfortunately, phrases I hear frequently are: "I only wear a little perfume, but it's all-natural, so it's okay," or "My perfume is very light, so it won't bother you." People often inform me that their personal products are different and, therefore, not offensive to me. I don't want to always tell everyone how wrong they are, but trust me. You are; *you are all wrong.*

My anger and frustration have made me less polite and less worried about offending anyone. I know that I can be pretty abrasive sometimes, and in those moments, I just don't care. Other people's fragrances can feel like an assault on me. And I'm nobody's victim anymore.

I also feel a need to give a voice to the unheard thirty percent who are sitting next to you on airplanes, in restaurants, and at weddings and events. The people who are too polite to tell you that you are making them sick, ruining their special moments with your secondhand fragrance. It's not just me that I am asking you to consider. I am asking you to think about who else you will impact next time you pick up that bottle of perfume, or wash your clothes in scented laundry products. You might not be thinking about them while you are enjoying your night out, but they are most certainly thinking about you.

I cannot truly understand what it's like for my hearing-impaired friends to be in a loud and crowded restaurant. I don't really know what it takes for someone who is mentally ill to get through each and every day. So, I don't expect anyone to totally *get* what my experience is when I'm around your "all-natural" and "light fragrances." But I do expect you to accept that my perception is my reality. And maybe, hopefully, after reading this book, more people will come to understand that by helping me and other people with allergies or sensitivities, you are *also* helping yourself and others that you care about.

Please know that I desperately want to be like any other person and just hang out with friends and family, go places, and travel without thinking about any of this stuff. But I can't. I just can't. Not yet anyway.

Most chemically sensitive people are struggling just to get through the day, or any situation, and don't always have the energy, confidence, or bandwidth to ask for special treatment. So many of them have never even been diagnosed with environmental illness or chemical sensitivity, so they don't even know the "rules" or how to help themselves.

Having an invisible chronic illness erodes self-confidence because you are so often the subject of other people's disbelief and disdain.

When we are suddenly under assault in a public place, we don't want to make a scene or make our companions uncomfortable with our strange and annoying requests. We are already all too aware that our family and friends are putting up with a lot more than they would like, and creating a scene might just be the straw that breaks the camel's back of a relationship.

It's easy to become withdrawn and reclusive. Little freedoms, like the ability to just go shopping and buy something new to wear, create a new look, or go to the salon, disappear little by little until suddenly, all of the daily small moments that you took for granted are miles away from manageable, and you start to lose yourself. You don't realize these things are an essential part of how you feel about yourself until you can't do them anymore. This translates into how we interact with our co-workers, friends, and family, and how our relationships with them are framed.

I never had to give a minute's thought to any of these things before I got sick. Then, in what felt like overnight, my life seemed to turn into an endless strategy session of how to navigate the world. It's one thing to figure it out for yourself, but if you have a spouse or a family, then they might as well be sick too. Dene can't smell what I am smelling, but I'm always expecting him to be sensitive to what is happening to me. Therefore, his life is easily nearly as restrictive as mine.

He *can* travel like a normal person if I'm not going on the trip, and get on a plane, stay in a hotel, rent a car, and visit with his friends who live in other states, go on business trips - just like a normal person. But when he comes home, he has to go through a complete decontamination process. His luggage and clothes go straight into the laundry room. I won't even talk to him until he showers off the stink of the airport, airplane, hotel, etc. He literally can't smell it at all, and for me, it's like being punched in the face the minute he walks in the door.

Dene is a very personable and outgoing guy who makes friends easily. But he knows he can't just bring a new friend home to hang out and watch a game if I have not vetted them out first. We've found ways to compromise so both of our needs are met. But I know sometimes it is incredibly frustrating to deal with me and all of the things that I expect him to be aware of on my behalf.

Meeting new friends was traditionally challenging for someone like me, who has always been shy, but now it is at a whole other level. Old friends are more forgiving, and if they value your friendship and care about you, they will make allowances for you. But I just couldn't spend time with people who were fragranced anymore, and I was tired of always being the fragrance police. New friends aren't typically interested in being given a list of changes they need to make if they want to be around you, and I was now worn out from asking family, friends, and employees to accommodate me over the years, so I tended not to try to make new friends.

This means my husband does not get to have many new friends either, for the same reasons. It just gets so complicated. Ironically though, for a couple of vegetarians, we have found that the easiest people for me to be around are often hunters. Hunters like to be fragrance-free so that the animals can't smell them coming. Sometimes the universe really has a sense of humor.

My family, most of whom live across the country, stays fragrance-free for me in case I ever come to visit or when they come to see me. They know it's something you have to work at and be consistent with, or I can't be around them. Of course, they also know that it's healthier for them and that by considering my needs, they are taking care of themselves, too. But they would not need to make it such a concentrated focus if it wasn't for me.

In case it's not apparent by now, chemically sensitive people can be *very* difficult to deal with. Dr. L told me that most chemically sensitive patients end up divorced. Dene and I really work on not adding to that statistic, but sometimes, it's really tough on him. Make that most of the time. When I am having an exposure, there are a lot of things happening behind the scenes that cause me to behave unpredictably or unpleasantly. For one thing, it affects my brain—a lot. It's different for everyone, but when chemically sensitive people are having an exposure, our brains just don't always work right.

For me, this presents in a lot of different ways. One way is I might start having difficulty finding words, and I'll start stuttering or just completely shut down verbally. If I've gotten to a place where I've shut down verbally, things are very bad, and I am no longer making good decisions. I depend on my family to notice I'm suddenly "not right" and get me out of the exposure. This happens when I'm trying to avoid ruining an event, and instead of saying I need to leave, I think I can suck it up and power through. But then somewhere in there, I'm no longer rational, and I am not able to recognize I need to get fresh air and that I am starting to be cognitively impaired by the exposure.

There's no question that I get jumpy and irritable when we go pretty much anywhere and I am having an exposure, or *even just think I'm about to have an exposure.* Instead of just enjoying the moment, I am strategizing to minimize my exposure and only giving a small part of my attention to who I am with or what we are doing. I'm just planning my exit strategy.

My impairment is often exacerbated by my tendency to use alcohol as a coping mechanism when I am in a place where I know I am about to be bombarded with fragrances and chemicals, but I don't want to be a party pooper and demand to leave. I don't want Dene or anyone else to have to stop having fun just because I'm special. So, I will sometimes use alcohol to get through a situation because even though I know I am still getting sick, alcohol will enable me to ignore it in the very short term.

I don't recommend this. It doesn't prevent you from getting sick; it just allows you to ignore that you are getting sick for a hot minute. When my brain is already not functioning correctly because of an exposure, dumping alcohol on the problem is foolish. It can even be dangerous, as chemically sensitive people can stroke out from a prolonged exposure. So yes, drinking my way through an exposure is downright idiotic, but sometimes I just don't give a shit because I *just want to feel normal*.

It's so hard always to be saying, "No I don't want to go out, or I can't go to your event." Eventually, people stop offering invitations, and the world gets even smaller. You worry your husband is becoming resentful, so you find ways to make it work, even when you know you are only making yourself sicker in the bigger picture. It's very lonely being chemically sensitive, but worse than that is knowing you are isolating the people you love the most.

Chemically sensitive people are sometimes just complete assholes. Myself included. Remember, when exposed to toxins, our brains don't work correctly. I have confronted complete strangers in restaurants and stores because of this. We can get belligerent with just about anyone once the brain is compromised and the filter disengages. I appreciate Dene and my family and friends so much for all their sacrifices, patience, and consideration. I'm not so sure that I would be as tolerant of myself and some of my behaviors as they have been. I am beyond blessed to have them in my life.

On the other hand, I am the canary in the coal mine for my people, and most of them recognize that by now. If I am complaining about someone's product, then not only is it not good for me, but it's also not good for them. Just because they are not having a reaction to it doesn't mean it's not affecting them. As annoying as I quite often am, my loved ones are also, at least sometimes, grateful to have a compass that shows them which products to avoid. They know that in the long run, if they follow my lead in avoiding certain products and being fragrance-free, they *will* be healthier.

CHAPTER 10

TIME FOR A NEW PLAN

I had been mindlessly following doctor's orders for years, and I was not cured. Indeed, things were improved, and I had regained some freedom, but I was not *free*, and still had many limitations. I used to believe medicine was more of an exact science, and I trusted that doctors had a plan for me based on known factors and predictable results. It was ingrained in me to trust them and follow the treatment plan without question, just as my mom had with her pregnancies.

As time went on, it became apparent to me that, although my environmental doctors certainly had a better handle on my problem than my traditional doctors, at some level, they were still just proceeding with a certain amount of trial and error. I'm not trying to imply it was all just guesswork. I'm just saying there was a lot of "try this and see how well you tolerate it."

I began to observe that they didn't really know what the end result of my treatment looked like because it's different for each environmentally ill patient. That's why they always wanted to do more testing and more testing again, followed by adjustments to my treatment, then more testing followed by more adjustments. It's great that they always worked towards an end goal of wellness for me, but…

I started to feel like an experiment.

To be crystal clear, they helped me a LOT, and I will always be grateful. If I had not found Dr. L, rather, if Dene had not found her for me, I would most certainly be dead by now, or worse. Continuing down a path of throwing drugs at the symptoms would have led to me likely having a stroke, being housebound, probably bedridden, chronic pain, and ultimately, I probably would have checked out. She truly saved my life. Also, to be fair, I will reiterate that every chronically ill patient is different and unique and requires a unique treatment plan. So it was great that I was *better*; I just started to lose faith that I was ever going to be *normal* again.

When I first started seeing the environmental doctors, I still didn't know what was wrong with me, what to do about it, or why it was happening. At least some of these questions were answered. They took the time to question and address *why* I had these symptoms and target the issue from multiple angles instead of just blindly prescribing drugs to mask or treat the individual symptoms. They recognized that I had a systemic problem that needed to be addressed in order to regain my health. My overall quality of life *had* improved dramatically.

But now I felt I had gone as far as I could with them. I was frustrated and weary. I had been so hopeful and confident, and now, years later, I was still waiting to be *cured*. Part of it was the money. I had spent a fortune on my treatment and was continuing to do so. I asked myself, how far would I take this if money was no object? And I realized that even if I had endless financial resources, which I most certainly did not, I would still be questioning the future of my treatment on this trajectory.

I was no longer confident in their ability to help make me *normal* again through the current treatment plan, as it had now been years. I had watched Yolanda Hadid on *Real Housewives of Beverly Hills* go to the ends of the earth for treatment of her mysterious chronic illness and struggle to reclaim her health. I'm sure her pockets are massively deeper than mine. If she couldn't find answers with her presumed big budget and worldwide contacts, how could I ever expect to be cured?

One of the things that Dr. L did that I really loved was that she gave me copies of every test result, every comment and observation she made, every single record, absolutely everything. This was so surprising to me, as up until that point, my doctors had always been the *keepers* of my information and would share results as they saw fit. Some of them clearly thought I was not intelligent or educated enough to understand my own medical records, or perhaps they considered these test results, notes, and records to be their intellectual property. Now I keep my own records, and I always ask for copies of lab and test results. After all, it's my life, my health, and my body; shouldn't I be in charge of or at least have access to the data?

I was no longer the same person who walked out of that doctor's office eight years prior crying and clutching a fistful of prescriptions, or the twenty-something who thought if she spoke up at the factory, she'd lose her job. That person was a victim and had been for most of her life. I was done with that.

I was not a victim anymore.

It was time to look for other solutions. I was frustrated from having gotten only so far with this treatment plan after not just spending a fortune funding it, but also having spent years of my life as its prisoner. I was now feeling well enough to be angry. I was pissed off at the circumstances that got me to that place—furious with the insurance companies for telling me to screw. I was angry at all the people in the world who continued to assault me and the planet with toxic chemicals. I wasn't just upset; I was enraged, irate, and fed up. I am an intelligent, capable woman. I was going to figure this out. I made the conscious decision to be my own advocate. Why shouldn't I be the one to determine which experiments to do on my own body? The insurance company considered it all an experiment, and at some point, I felt like that too. I was tired of being stuck.

Slowly, I eliminated parts of my treatment. I wanted to see what would happen, what was *really* working for me, and what was *not*. I wanted to get back to just me and my body and see what would happen. I would still be fragrance-free, eat organic, and be mindful of exposures, but I was done taking all of the drugs, supplements, and injections. So, I simply stopped.

An interesting thing happened. Nothing. *Nothing happened.* I had stopped everything, and I was okay-ish. I was not cured; I still had issues, but *I did not get worse!* This was huge for me. Minimally, it seemed like if I discontinued the treatments that seemed to have stalled, I would not lose any ground that I had so painstakingly gained. I started to believe in my own ability to change things independently. Just to be clear, I'm not saying that all of those treatments never did me any good-they most certainly did. But I had now determined that I was no longer making forward progress.

Through internet research, I stumbled across a program called the Dynamic Neural Retraining System (DNRS). It turns out that DNRS was founded by a chemically sensitive person, and she has numerous videos from other chemically sensitive people claiming the DNRS program had improved their lives or even cured them. Of course, I immediately bought the program and dove right in.

The premise of DNRS is that chemical sensitivity is caused by a brain injury in which the brain's limbic system - part of the autonomic nervous system – *remember the tilt table test?* - becomes impaired and can no longer distinguish between actual danger and everyday chemicals. The program guides you through daily practices designed to retrain your brain through various meditations and exercises so that the limbic system no longer sees common chemicals as a level-ten threat. The plan utilizes the brain's inherent plasticity to correct and re-wire.

Maybe this was going to be the thing that would finally cure me all the way! I was very excited about it, especially since I knew that I had actual physical brain injuries and lesions from a fall - *remember the 99 restaurant?* I also knew that my autonomic nervous system was dysfunctional. I have dysautonomia. I was not discounting everything I had learned from the environmental doctors, but now I was thinking that my brain injury was a factor as well. I had a new path forward. Again.

I went all in on the DNRS plan for about a year, and I did see some additional improvement in my sensitivities, but then I plateaued with this program as well. The good news is that I was in a better place than when I started. In addition, I was gaining confidence in my ability to find my own way to being "cured." I also learned a lot about brain plasticity and the importance of having a positive attitude. This was the very beginning of my understanding that *thoughts matter*, and an adjustment in my perspective of *my* role in my recovery.

Back then, I was only touching on the edges of this concept, but it was the start of a fundamental shift in how I viewed myself and the world around me. I had only recently developed the self-awareness that I had spent most of my life in a victim mentality. Now, I was actively deciding that not only was I *not a victim*, I was also *not a sick person*. I was not broken or unfixable; in fact, I could choose to focus on how good I felt.

I had gained a lot of weight during my treatment, and I was determined to deal with that now as well. I started eating a little healthier, walking my dogs, exercising at home, and I lost about twenty pounds. This was encouraging, so I signed up for a weight-loss program at my chiropractor's office and lost about another forty pounds.

I was living a much more normal life now. I no longer had pain all of the time. The headaches were relatively infrequent, and when they did show up, did not last more than a day or so. I was able to be around some fragrances or even cleaning products for short periods of time without having symptoms. My skin looked good again, and I actually felt pretty good a lot of the time. However, since I was still unable to tolerate laundry products and certain fragrances and chemicals. My freedom and, consequently, Dene's freedom to some degree, continued to be limited.

I was still searching for my ultimate cure, and I read a lot of books in my quest. In 2018, I stumbled across *Liver Rescue by Anthony William*. This book discusses the functions of the liver and gives recommendations on how to cleanse your liver so that your body operates better overall. Remember Medical Medium, who told me all those years ago that I was full of toxins? I had totally forgotten about him, but this was his book!

I found the notes from my consultation with him years prior. I realized that much of what he had told me, and what was in this book, corroborated both what the acupuncturist had said, as well as environmental medicine's bucket theory. I decided to do the ten-day liver cleanse recommended in the book. My fabulous, supportive husband agreed to do it with me. The cleanse was basically a vegan, whole-food diet with certain restrictions and a focus on a high intake of certain fruits and vegetables that would help purge toxins.

We both felt like crap at first, but I already knew from experience that detoxing will do that to you. We followed the cleanse to the letter, and for the first several days, neither of us was having a good time, but we persevered. At the end of the nine days, we observed that we both felt good — *really* good. We decided to take it to thirty days just to see what would happen. At the end of the thirty days, the results were undeniable.

Dene commented that he felt better than he had in decades, and I was noticing changes and improvement as well. We knew it was not realistic to stay on this strict liver cleanse, but we picked it apart to see what we thought were the most important aspects that we could realistically maintain. We formulated a plan of eating a gluten-free, organic, vegan, whole-food diet high in fruits and vegetables and low in grains. We gave up meat, seafood, alcohol, eggs, dairy, and canola oil. When I did buy processed food (which was rare), I made sure it was free of "natural flavorings," which, of course, are just another form of chemicals most of the time.

We drank celery juice every morning and worked out three

times a week with a trainer. Over the next year, I lost about another 40 pounds, for a total weight loss of about 100 pounds. At my heaviest, I had ballooned up to about 265 pounds. Now back to 165 for the first time in many years, I was at a weight that felt healthy and right for me. I almost felt like a normal person again. Suddenly, I was able to go into stores or restaurants without dire consequences. I still struggled with laundry fragrances and personal products containing certain chemicals, like hairspray, sunscreen, or some highly fragranced products. But I was *significantly* better than I had been for years. I could see the light at the end of the tunnel.

I started to believe I really would be able to be completely cured. My husband also reaped the rewards of our new healthy eating plan, feeling good and having improved health. We agreed that plant-based was the way to go for us and committed to that choice. Some unexpected things happened after that.

After about six months, I noticed a change in my attitude. Or rather, more subtly, a change in how I viewed life. I had spent my entire life being a fearful person. Part of it, I think, was unwittingly taught to me by my well-intended mother and grandmother. This seems a little counterintuitive because they were both very strong women. But I realized many of my earliest memories were of them sharing their fears with me, which I then adopted as my own. But my overall fearfulness predominantly seemed to come naturally, as if I was born that way. My family used to say, "Oh, she's just bashful."

The truth was that as a child, and then later still as a teenager, I was terrified of nearly everything. Most of my earliest memories involve me being afraid of something or someone. I was scared of dogs (even though I wanted a puppy more than anything, but that's another story.) I was afraid of strangers, not just shy, but terrified. I was fearful of new places and new things, the unknown. I was afraid of school, the other kids, the teachers, adults, the potential for failure. As I got older, I excelled at hiding my fears. I had learned that some people will use your fear as a weapon against you. But behind the facade, I was very fearful and, truth be told, secretly depressed.

My deepest, darkest secret since I was a very young child was that I contemplated suicide daily. I never shared that with anyone because I did not want to be watched and potentially stopped if I ever decided to go through with it. But it was always in the back of my mind and at times, very much in the front. As a child, I was having thoughts of suicide before I was even old enough to understand what it was or how to do it. The thing that always kept me in check was I understood how much it would hurt the people I loved if I were to act on those thoughts, and that was not acceptable. I spent so much of my young life being fearful and depressed and hiding that from everyone, by the time I was an adult, I was an expert at pretending I was okay.

After about six months of being strictly plant-based, I began to notice that I was not as fearful and depressed anymore. I actually felt happy most of the time. I *had* consciously been practicing being more positive for a little while now. But this felt bigger than that. I could not explain it.

Then, I stumbled upon a YouTube video in which a doctor talks about what happens when we eat animals. I don't recall her name and can't locate the video now, but her message really stuck with me. She pointed out that most animal products produced in the U.S.come from animals raised in feedlots and factory farms. These animals spend their entire lives in pain and misery, and then their last moments are spent in terror and pain. Their fear and pain are released into their bloodstream as hormones and spread throughout their bodies, which infiltrates the meat we eat or the dairy products we consume.

Suddenly, I made the connection that for nearly my entire life, I had been saturating my own body with the pain and fears of the animals that I had been eating. In fact, since I was an infant and had been fed *meat formula* instead of breast milk, it truly was literally my *entire* life that this had been happening.

Before you start telling me hormones that I eat from animals can't affect me like that, let me point out that there are multiple hormone therapies that are taken orally that are derived from animal sources. So clearly, we *can* eat animal hormones and have it affect us. I myself have been prescribed "Armour Thyroid," which is a pill that is taken orally and prescribed for certain thyroid conditions. It is derived from desiccated pig thyroid glands. So I ask you, what is the difference between that and all of the fear and pain hormones raging around in the same pig if I eat it? Or a cow, or a chicken? If I was eating all those fear and pain hormones from practically the day I was born, I don't see how it would *not* affect me.

It wasn't like I randomly decided that animal products made me fearful, and then I gave them up. It was the other way around. I had given up animal products and, after a period of time, came to notice that I was different, changed. Not only was I no longer fearful, but I also no longer thought about suicide or felt depressed. I now found it easy to have a positive attitude and intentions most of the time. Outwardly, most people probably would not have noticed a difference — I had become such an expert at hiding my thoughts and feelings behind an invisible suit of armor. But on the *inside*, it was a revelation.

Another thing happened that both Dene and I observed after several years of eating plant-based. We no longer got sick. I'm not talking about my chemical sensitivity, which was vastly improved even though not eliminated; I'm talking about the usual stuff, like colds, flus, and sore throats. In fact, after we went plant-based, we went years at a time without even catching a cold.

It was only very recently that Dene and I allowed ourselves to reintegrate dairy products when we were eating out. After "falling off the cheese wagon" we both got sick twice. First, with some kind of bug, and then Covid finally caught up with us this winter. Coincidence?

After Dene and I had been plant-based for nearly a year, we stumbled across *The Game Changers* on Netflix. It's a documentary created by James Cameron, Arnold Schwarzenegger, and Jackie Chan. The film is about professional fighter James Wilks, who gets injured and is searching for ways to heal faster. He stumbles across information claiming that the ancient Roman gladiators were mainly plant-based because it helped them heal faster, so he embarks on a quest for more information about how our food affects our health, healing, and performance.

The film is excellent, and Dene and I found it corroborated what we had already recently discovered about being plant-based. We not only felt better, but there were measurable improvements to our health, including cholesterol, blood pressure, weight, and skin appearance. My sensitivities were improved, and of course the aforementioned changes I felt emotionally and mentally. I was profoundly changed. We were fully committed to a permanent plant-based lifestyle, which was now a big part of my new treatment plan.

I now had new tools again. I was eating plant-based all the time and organic as much as possible. In deciding to take care of my liver and assist it in processing toxins, I gave up drinking alcohol. I was using my thoughts to retrain my brain and, consequently, no longer identified as a sick person.

I was genuinely reclaiming my life.

CHAPTER 11

THOUGHTS MATTER

There are a number of things I think would be very different now if I had never gotten sick.

For years, you could not have convinced me under any condition that something good could come from my chronic illness. It was so difficult and so painful for so long; I only wanted it to end, and wished it had never happened to me. Over time, however, my perspective has changed, and now I believe good things have come from it.

I love being a vegetarian. Funny how it was something that I wanted to do more than once when I was younger, and finding my way there was not a straight path by any means, but this is where I wound up after all. Notice I said vegetarian and not vegan? I try to be vegan; I really do. But now that I am healthy enough to go out occasionally, I love being able to go out to a restaurant with my husband like a *normal* person. I love not having to shop for and cook every single bite of food I put in my mouth. Maybe that doesn't sound like a big deal, but it is to me. Sometimes, I just want to take a break or feel a little pampered.

We live in New Mexico now, and the cuisine here is not

exactly known for being vegan-friendly. A disproportionately large percentage of the meatless options here have cheese in them. (I'm looking at YOU cheese enchiladas and chile rellenos.) Yes, cheese is my downfall when eating out, and I freely admit it. I try to avoid it most of the time though, and think of it as a special treat. I also try to be very discerning with where the cheese is sourced if I do choose to serve it at home—only organic, grass-fed, pasture-raised is acceptable if I am buying cheese for home, which I generally only do when we are having guests. When I do eat cheese, I think about the sacrifice of the animals involved in making it and offer them my gratitude and respect. So, I'm vegan about 90% of the time, and the other 10% I'm vegetarian. I'm good with that for now. I would like to be 100% plant-based again, and I definitely go through very long periods with no cheese, but I find it very hard to keep that up when we go out.

We don't watch violent television or movies anymore. Dene and I consciously look for programming skewed towards or embracing positivity, like *Ted Lasso* on AppleTV or *The Curse of Oak Island* on the History Channel. I love focusing our time and attention on shows and entertainment that highlight positive people, kindness, and respect. It is no longer acceptable for us to watch shows that feature murder as entertainment. We are more discerning and thoughtful about our choices now. Violence needs to be germane to the plot, or we find it distracting, unnecessary, and distasteful. If we choose to watch something that suddenly takes a turn into being too dark, we stop watching it.

I have already confessed to being a *Real Housewives* fan. I love to see the fashions, and the closets of the ladies, but more importantly, I have learned from these women that we should never give up hope, and never say never. I have watched long enough that I have seen women who you would think could not even be in a room together in a million years suddenly find a way to forgive each other and become friends again. Don't get me wrong, I know that the producers stage these scenarios for dramatic effect, but that doesn't mean that real feelings can't be hurt, actual damage done, and ultimately, old friends or family members forgiven. I find that to be weirdly comforting and inspiring despite all of the other negative bullshit that goes on in those shows.

Being selective about what we expose ourselves to is a big deal to us now. We consciously choose to surround ourselves with positive people and situations. Ironically, while we are actively doing that, I have observed some of the people in our lives who lean towards the negative actively weed us out first! It seems that vibrationally when we mismatch, we naturally drift apart.

I'm not perfect at any of this, but I'm better than I ever have been. I genuinely believe it is making a difference in how I feel and my overall quality of life.

Multiple avenues led me to the concept that thoughts matter—so many, in fact, that I had to take it seriously. When you have a chronic illness, you find yourself spending a lot of time with your best friends, Google, and YouTube, searching for answers. And sometimes, you find yourself wandering down some unexpected rabbit holes.

The first time I saw a video of Dr. Joe Dispenza talking about using his brain to overcome paralysis from his accident, I was entranced. If brain plasticity worked for him, then it could work for me, right?

Or what about Abraham-Hicks, an extra-dimensional being/ collective channeled through Esther Hicks? I was fascinated by Abraham's teaching of the Law of Attraction. I was learning that we create our own reality, that we manifest what we think about. It does not matter if you are thinking about what you do want or what you don't want, because if you are thinking about it, then you are drawing it to you.

I do not believe I would have found my way to these teachers and learned these concepts if I had not been searching for answers to my illness. I love that this path has brought me to understand that **being happy is a choice.** This is so fundamentally important that it bears repeating. **Happiness is a choice.** It's that simple.

No matter how bleak or challenging a day may be, *we choose the place from which we are going to receive it,* and, consequently, how we will interact with or react to it. No one else is responsible for my happiness. I love my husband, and I am grateful for him in my life, but he does not *make me happy*; only I can do that. It is *my* choice.

In June of 2021, Jane Marczewski, AKA Nightbirde, performed during the 16th season auditions on America's Got Talent. If you haven't seen a clip of that audition, then you should stop reading this and Google it immediately. Spoiler alert: she bangs out a beautiful original song despite the fact that she had been battling cancer and been given a 2% chance of survival. After she's done singing, she tells the judges, *"You can't wait until life isn't hard anymore until you decide to be happy."* And she said, *"2% is not zero."* In less than ten minutes, this tiny wisp of a woman affected the lives of millions of people because she understood fundamentally that happiness is a choice. Her remarkable display of resilience and wisdom resonated globally, inspiring countless individuals, including me.

I have spent so much of my life being fearful, depressed, and helpless. I honestly thought that things happened to me because of luck or chance, and I would *react*, not *respond*. I had no idea that I could *choose* to respond in a positive way regardless of what the situation was. I used to *expect* to react to negative stimuli with fear, depression, or anger. It never even remotely occurred to me that it was *always* my choice how to respond and not just react. Knowing now that it is and always has been my choice, is a gift more precious than any cure.

A TED Talk I saw on YouTube discussed what happens when we are presented with a situation that makes us angry or fearful. Our bodies release hormones in response to events, which are what make us feel angry or afraid. These reactions are a kneejerk, physiological response. However, most of these hormones will naturally dissipate within twenty minutes. This means that after that initial reaction, you are now *choosing* how you want to respond. This is a pretty simplistic way to look at it, but fundamentally, what is important to note is that we *choose* how we feel, even when it seems like we are a victim of circumstance.

Every day when I get up in the morning now, I consciously decide that it's going to be a great day — no matter what lies in my path. I *consciously* decide that I am happy, regardless of what else is happening all around me. Dene and I actively choose to spend our time with other people who feel the same way. Do I feel better physically because I have mentally decided that I feel better? Yes, no question about it. Is it a great day because I have decided that it's a great day? Absolutely it is, no question about it.

Of course, there are still challenges to overcome. But now I look at challenges as simply that-challenges, and as I overcome them, I am stronger and better. I would not trade my newfound belief and understanding of this fundamental truth for anything, not even a magic pill to cure me. This is a life-changing gift that I do not believe I would have discovered without having become chronically ill.

My illness has literally given me the gift of happiness. There is no other way to see it. In my search for a cure, I learned something so much more important: I learned how to be happy, no matter what.

My mother died in September of 2021, after a long and difficult battle with Alzheimer's. I was already on my way to see her that morning when the hospice nurse called to tell me she was transitioning. As I drove the ninety minutes to visit with her, knowing it might be her last day on Earth, I still made the decision that it was going to be a great day. My brother, my dad, and I were there with her when she passed. Of course, it was emotional and painful, and of course, I still miss her terribly. But I am grateful that she was not alone when she went. She knew we were there with her and that we were going to be okay and be strong for each other and the rest of the family. She was able to let go and pass on peacefully and gracefully; surrounded by love.

Making the decision and setting my intention that morning that I was going to be happy and that it would be a great day was the behavior of the person that I now was, *not* the fearful victim that I had spent my life being. This allowed me to accept her passing with the love and grace that was worthy of her, which was the best thing I could do for her in her final moments.

This was a gift that my illness had given me. The person that I had been ten years before, and quite frankly, my whole life before that, was fearful and depressed. That person would have found a way to be a victim of Mom's passing. That person would not have allowed Mom to go peacefully and gracefully but likely would have made it all about *me* due to a lack of self-confidence and fear. My illness had been transformative for me but in such an unexpected way. Without it, I would never have grown in the way that my mom needed when Alzheimer's struck.

I am grateful for all the lessons and catalysts that my chronic illness has provided. Of course, I'd love to release the chains completely and have total freedom of movement, travel, and social interaction with no concern or thought of physical repercussions; with no pain or discomfort due to exposures. Thanks, Universe; I'm all set now! But would I trade my new-found happiness and clarity for health and physical freedom? Nope, not for anything.

• • •

I had never really thought about whether it mattered what I was thinking. I'd often heard the expression, "Don't even put that out to the universe" or similar, or even used it myself, kind of like "knock on wood." But I had always just assumed that my thoughts are my own, and as long as I don't say it out loud, and am keeping it to myself, then there is no impact anywhere. I no longer believe this.

Science is consistently proving that thought does matter, or rather, that everything is connected. Consider the Quantum Mechanics Double-Slit Experiment. While not precisely or directly an experiment about human thought, it explores the role of observation in quantum mechanics, specifically the behavior of particles when they are observed. The results indicate a "connection" between the observer and the observed and prove that *the act of observing affects the outcome of the experiment.* Cleve Backster's plant experiments proved that plants would "react" to human thought. He observed that a polygraph instrument attached to a plant would record that the plant registered a change in electrical resistance when it was threatened with harm. In other words, he proved that *a plant would react to human thought.*

Perhaps the most well-known demonstration of the effects of thoughts are the water experiments performed by Dr. Masaru Emoto. Using high-speed photographs and magnetic resonance analysis, Dr. Emoto *scientifically proved that water reacts to human intention.*

Specifically, water exposed to loving, benevolent, and compassionate intentions would present physical molecular formations in shapes generally considered pleasing, balanced, and attractive. Conversely, water exposed to fearful and negative human emotions responded by presenting shapes that we would generally consider to be unbalanced, discordant, and unattractive.

His experiments included proving that the polluted and toxic water from the Fujiwara Dam actually changed its shape at a molecular level from distorted and unbalanced to a balanced crystalline pattern when exposed to Buddhist prayer. Dr. Emoto is considered a pioneer in this field, and scientists continue to build upon his work with fascinating results, some of which have practical applications.

How is this relevant to my health issues? Our bodies are mainly composed of water. Therefore, how could thought *not* affect us? If positive and loving thought changes the shape of water at a molecular level, and we are mainly composed of water, then therefore doesn't it stand to reason that positive or negative thought will similarly affect us? How could it not? And what does it cost you to try?

Many sources currently cite the "Law of Attraction" and one of its fundamental aspects: manifestation. These concepts are generally framed within the broader context of what is considered the "New Thought" movement, which includes various spiritual and philosophical beliefs centered around the power of the mind. Although sometimes controversial and not universally scientifically accepted, there is growing evidence that supports certain aspects of these concepts.

Basically, the Law of Attraction states that *like attracts like, and therefore, positive or negative thoughts will correspondingly attract positive or negative experiences into a person's life.* There is an enormous amount of material available on this and similar subjects, but I'd like to share some of the ways I think it is relevant to my story.

I talk about some of the things that happened because of my illness that I am grateful for. Becoming a vegetarian, living a positive lifestyle, letting go of my victim mentality, becoming fearless, and learning to *choose to be happy.* Even learning about the Law of Attraction and manifestation would not have happened if I had not been searching for a cure for my illness.

The person I am today, who I like to think of as much more positive, grateful, and happy, would not exist if I had never gotten sick. I love the person I am today, and I believe that the road for me to manifest the life that I have now was largely formed in the cauldron of my years of chronic illness and the path I chose to find my way out.

There is no way of knowing what person I would have become without the catalyst of my illness, but I am reasonably sure I would not like her very much. Her life would be sad, full of fear and anger, perhaps comparatively short, and undoubtedly miserable. She would be a helpless and depressed victim. They say the universe works in mysterious ways, and it is unfolding in the way it is meant to. I do wholeheartedly believe that to be true, and find it comforting.

When I met my first environmental doctor and received a diagnosis, I was incredibly relieved. I finally had an explanation; I could now *prove* to people that it was not all in my head. I expected that my problems were about to be over. This doctor helped me a great deal, and I believe saved my life. All of which I am, of course, extremely grateful for. She *also* reconfirmed to me how ill I was. Instead of encouraging me to think like a healthy person, she said, "You are a very sick woman."

I realize now I internalized that, embraced it, and I got *worse* before I got better. There were many factors involved, including unmasking and detoxing, but certainly, one factor being what was going on in my head. Having a doctor say that reinforced my victim mentality and indirectly, or perhaps directly, influenced my state of being.

She told me I was very sick, and so I was. I now *identified* as a sick person, and my world got even smaller. To be clear, I'm not suggesting that she "thought me into being sick," or that I "thought myself sick," or that it was all in my head either. Nor was she trying to brainwash me into needing treatment.

The point I'm making is that in addition to the physiological events that were happening due to my numerous toxic exposures, a layer of complexity was added: a negative state of mind and being. I had consciously decided that I was, in fact, a very sick woman — just like the doctor said. This *had* to be affecting my overall well-being, but at the time, I had no clue.

This is an area of great inner conflict for me. Although I had been physically struggling for years and was at the end of my rope, up until that moment, no doctor had *validated* my illness. By just feeding me prescriptions to treat my symptoms, they never really acknowledged that I was chronically ill. Dr. L telling me how sick I was actually shifted my perception of my reality. This changed how I thought of myself. I went from thinking of myself as just a random collection of symptoms to being "a very sick woman."

I realize that she was just trying to get me to take my diagnosis and treatment plan seriously. She knew it was going to be an expensive and difficult road, and that I was unlikely to engage in treatment if I didn't think I needed it. I knew I was ill, but now I had someone of authority, *a doctor*, confirming it and telling me how *serious* it was. I'm not saying that my condition wasn't serious; it very much was. I'm just making the observation that, at that point, I was encouraged to think of myself as very ill, and that affected how I identified myself and, consequently, how I navigated life for years to come.

I will never know which parts of my treatment helped me, which parts were superfluous, or how much of my suffering was exacerbated by my mental state and my perception of the state of my health. I trust that the universe is unfolding in the way it is meant to, and that includes me getting sick and then finding my way back to "normal" or perhaps never being completely cured. But I also truly believe that a critical factor in turning the tide eventually came from *within* myself. Conversely, when I was at my sickest was also when I totally embraced that I was gravely ill, and so it was true.

I am certainly not suggesting that you can wish illness away. I'm not saying that if you have cancer, all you need to do is think of yourself as a healthy person, and it will disappear. I *am* saying that how you perceive yourself *is as important as the rest of your treatment.* The "power of positive thinking" is not bullshit. It is real and should be taken seriously. I have experienced this firsthand and will never doubt it again.

I'm also not suggesting that doctors should never tell someone they are sick. I'm only making the observation that, for me, when I suddenly had permission to wallow in it, I believe the Law of Attraction reacted in kind. I allowed my diagnosis to become part of my *identity.* And, as I sat in those treatment centers with the other patients and thought, "I don't want to end up like that" over and over, I now believe I was literally aligning myself with that reality and drawing it to me.

In the context of the Law of Attraction, it has been said to me that "irritation attracts more irritation." I have found it to be essential to manage my exposures without becoming "irritated." This is tricky since the nature of an exposure generally causes me some sort of physical pain or irritation. Earlier on, as you may have noticed, I was quite angry and did myself a disservice by indulging in negative emotions as a result of an exposure.

Now, I find that if I can manage to leave the negative emotions out of it and focus on what is positive around me, it's much easier to navigate an exposure incident. Sure, I still hide in my house when my neighbors are doing laundry, but I don't obsess over whether or not I should confront them or consider gifting them with a basket of fragrance-free laundry products. I simply remove myself from the problem while it is happening and move on to something else.

I have observed that even the act of writing this book has caused me to backslide a little. I have worked hard to look to the future and not dwell in the past. There are so many details that I have put behind me or tried to forget; so much of it seems like it was just a bad dream. Focusing on what happened and how I felt so I can document it here and share it has been a struggle and brings me back a little too much. I have worked hard not to identify as just a chemically sensitive person, so I have found it uncomfortable to write those words multiple times in this book.

You may have noticed that I have often jumped back and forth between first and second person in this book. I found myself doing it unconsciously because I now choose to *not* relate as a sick person or as chemically sensitive. When I talk about it in first person, it pulls me back to the place I have worked so hard to put behind me. It's easier, or safer rather, for me to project these struggles on You, (sorry) and share my thoughts as if You are the sick one, rather than presenting *every* thought as a Me thing or a Me struggle.

I am committed to sharing my journey because I understand what it's like to feel helpless and alone when your doctor doesn't know how to help. Over the past several years, whenever I've shared even a small piece of what I've learned, people have wanted to know more—because they, or someone they love, have experienced something similar. It's important to me to take everything I've been through and everything I've learned and present it in a cohesive way so that others might find something useful for their own journeys. Now that you know how I arrived here and what my life has been like, let's dive into some facts.

CHAPTER 12

AMERICA'S OBSESSION WITH FRAGRANCE

I now cannot imagine working for someone else and being subjected to the fragrances and chemicals on other people or in the workplace, whether it be cleaning products or carpets, fragrances or whatever. No one should be put in that situation.

In 2006, a woman filed a complaint and successfully sued the city of Detroit for not providing a fragrance-free workplace. In *McBride v. City of Detroit,* senior city planner Susan McBride was awarded $100,000, and the city agreed to revise its ADA handbook and training and post notices about the fragrance-free policy.

McBride, who is chemically sensitive, voiced complaints after a colleague began wearing strong perfume and utilized a room deodorizer at the workplace. Although the coworker ceased using the deodorizer at McBride's request, she continued to wear the perfume. McBride sought assistance from her supervisor and the human resources department, only to be told by the city that her colleague had a *constitutional* right to wear perfume and that, because McBride was the one with the affliction, it was her issue to deal with, not the employers. The federal judiciary, however, held a different view. It determined that being allergic to fragrances could qualify as a disability under the ADAAA, which is enforced by the Equal Employment Opportunity Commission (EEOC). According to this ruling, severe reactions to odors or scents classify as disabilities. The ruling emphasized that once an individual is allergic to a substance, increasingly minimal amounts can trigger these symptoms. Ultimately, the court recognized McBride's Multiple Chemical Sensitivity, or MCS, as a disability that significantly hindered her essential life function of breathing.

Then there is *Wilbert Bazert v. State of Louisiana.* Wilbert Bazert was employed by the Department of Corrections at a Louisiana State Penitentiary for sixteen years until May 1995, at which time he was transferred to another part of the prison that increased his exposure to cleaning products, fragrances, personal products, and cigarette smoke.

Due to the effect of these secondhand fragrances and smoke on his asthma, he requested and subsequently was denied a transfer. The trial court rendered judgment in favor of Wilbert Bazert and awarded him $150,000.00 in damages and $29,370 in interest and attorney's fees. Additionally, the court ordered that he be reinstated in his original position with back pay and that all of his annual and sick leave be restored.

There are other cases, but the point is this: We do have rights, *and there are legal precedents establishing that chemical sensitivity, MCS and or asthma, qualify as disabilities and we have rights, which are enforceable.*

Why is it so hard to find good fragrance-free products? When did people start to think that a place or a thing has to smell like fruit or pine trees or it's not clean, whether that be our hair, floors, cars, clothing, or just about everything? When I was a child, not everything had a fragrance. At some point when I was a teenager, the myth about using dryer sheets to keep mosquitoes away started to circulate. That was followed by advice to put dryer sheets in your furniture drawers to keep everything "fresh" and put them in your empty suitcases or any place that needed to be "freshened up." Why does everything have to have a "fresh" scent, and what the hell exactly is a "fresh" scent anyway?

This was brilliant marketing by the dryer sheet companies, but it's all Bullshit. There is no scientific evidence to support the mosquito claim, and what is the deal with fooling ourselves by masking one odor with another? If your luggage smells bad because it's dirty or mildewy, then making it *also* smell like fake "fresh linen" isn't going to make your luggage suddenly be *clean* or not have mildew; instead it just has more toxic chemicals layered on top of the original stink and any toxic substances it picked up in airplanes, hotels, or your garage.

Quite frankly, I find it insulting to my intelligence to imply that I think something is clean just because it's covered in fragrance. Secondhand fragrance is not given the same consideration as secondhand cigarette or cigar smoke. It is now generally recognized pretty much everywhere in the U.S. that secondhand smoke is a real hazard that can cause cancer, heart attacks, and other health issues, and smokers are expected to keep to designated areas. If you are not a smoker and you don't want to breathe it, then you can usually avoid the places where it is still allowed. It took a long time for non-smokers to assert their rights to clean air in the fight against Big Tobacco, and now here we are yet again, and this time it's even more difficult.

So why is secondhand fragrance not considered pollution? It's easily as toxic and obnoxious as cigarette smoke. Is it because it's invisible? When I was at my sickest, I often felt like I could almost see it. I certainly could taste it. This is not surprising since our sense of taste is very much derived from what we are smelling. I don't understand how everyone accepts that secondhand smoke infringes on the rights of non-smokers, but that secondhand fragrance does not. Isn't the fundamental principle that we all have a right to breathe clean air the same?

How is it possible that so many people douse themselves in a toxic soup, inflict it on innocent bystanders, and nobody questions it? Why don't I have the same rights as the people who don't want to breathe secondhand smoke? Susan McBride and Wilbert Bazert have paved the way for employee rights, but what about the rest of us?

Where do we even begin? I suppose the first people who worked to make smoking in public places illegal felt like they were up against similar odds because smoking was so widely accepted at the time. It's Big Tobacco all over again, only now it's Big Chemical, and unfortunately, millions of people will continue to struggle and get sick. Some of them will even die before we can change this dynamic.

My environmental doctors told me that over thirty percent of the general population is chemically sensitive but undiagnosed, and that is considered a low estimate. Studies done between 2002-2006 *(Caress SM, Steinemann AC. Prevalence of fragrance sensitivity in the American population. J Environ Health. 2009 Mar;71(7):46-50. PMID: 19326669.)* asked test subjects if they found being next to someone wearing a fragrance to be attractive or irritating. Results showed that over thirty percent of the participants in the study found scented products on other people in their proximity irritating, with a large portion of these people experiencing either adverse health effects and/or irritation from secondhand fragrance, laundry product pollution, air fresheners, etc.

There is a well-established dynamic that it is not polite, or more accurately, it is considered *very offensive* to give negative feedback to someone about what they or their home smells like. Positive feedback is welcome all day long, but if the people who think you smell like hell because of your laundry and/or perfume never tell you, then you just blissfully and ignorantly go through life thinking you smell good. I am here to tell you that three out of ten people that you encounter every single day find the fragrances you have chosen to apply to yourself to be offensive and may even make them sick, but they are too polite to say anything. I'm not too polite. I'm telling you: You smell like hell, and you are making me sick.

Fragrance is *everywhere*. The average person is oblivious to the amount of toxic chemicals they randomly off-gas and inflict on the world around them. If you don't think fragrances and/or laundry products are toxic, don't just take my word for it, Google it, I dare you. Google: "Are fragrances Toxic?" You could spend a lifetime reading the thousands of articles, reports, research, and studies that will come up. If I cited them all here this book would be multiple volumes.

When I meet new people, if I try to talk to them about it, their eyes glaze over, and I can see them trying to decide if they are going to categorize me as a complete lunatic or just annoying. It's exhausting constantly being hyper-focused on something that is invisible to so many people, but that my health and very life depend on managing carefully.

Because fragrance is considered proprietary information or a trade secret, companies are not required to list the ingredients of a fragrance on a label. They only need to list "fragrance" as an ingredient. The problem is there are thousands of components used in fragrances, many of which are universally recognized as carcinogenic or toxic. As of the time of this writing, I have been unable to find any evidence of federal authorities regulating the safety of ingredients in fragrances, and so far, only baby steps at the state level, with the state of California having recently passed California Cosmetic Fragrance and Flavor Ingredient Right to Know Act of 2020.

At the federal level H.R. 5538 Cosmetic Fragrance and Flavor Ingredient Right to Know Act of 2021 was introduced in October of 2021. It was referred to the House Energy and Commerce Subcommittee on Health, and then…crickets. I recently contacted the office of Representative Janice D. Schakowsky from Illinois, who submitted the Bill, but have not received any new information or updates.

There are also HR 3619: The Toxic-Free Beauty Act (authored by Reps. Schakowsky & Fletcher), HR 3620: Cosmetic Safety for Communities of Color and Salon Workers (Reps. Schakowsky & Blunt Rochester), HR 3621: Cosmetic Fragrance and Flavor Right to Know Act (Reps. Schakowsky & Matsui), and HR 3622: Cosmetic Supply Chain Transparency Act (Rep. Schakowsky).

You can help by going to *safecosmetics.org*, a program of Breast Cancer Prevention Partners, and following the "take action" links to write letters to Congress or donate to the cause.

Another factor that skews the public perception of the safety of certain chemicals and correspondingly, the products they are used in, is that toxicological research is typically done on one chemical at a time for a specified amount of time. But, the average fragrance consists of dozens or more often even hundreds of chemicals, and the average person has multiple fragranced products on them or in their environment at any given time, and often for extended periods of time, or even all of the time. Since every person's personal chemical exposure is unique, then how can it possibly be determined that these products are safe for everyone? It is unrealistic for tests to have been performed that incorporate all the possible combinations of chemicals on any one person at any given time for their specific length of exposure.

Did you know that the fragrance industry is largely self-regulated? Some of my environmental doctors also shared with me that many fragrances have ingredients with narcotic-like qualities. Fragrances cross the blood-brain barrier, which usually shields our brains from toxic substances. The chemicals in these products can affect and manipulate our brains to want and desire more of these smells, even when we know it might be bad for us. There is a word for this; it's called addiction. See the article by John P. Thomas, *Health Impact News: The Addictive Power of Toxic Perfumes and Colognes: maskedcanaries.wordpress.com.*

The skin is the body's largest organ. Whatever you wash your clothes in infiltrates those fabrics and, consequently, infiltrates your skin when you wear those garments. On top of that, laundry fragrances are designed to be *sticky.* They advertise and promote how long the smell will last. Fascinatingly, the laundry product companies actually promote their "free and clear" or "sensitive care" products as "the safer choice" or "free of irritating dyes and perfumes." Doesn't that imply that they know and admit that their fragranced products are not a safe choice or that they can be irritating?

Because people can be addicted to their fragranced products, they are very resistant to giving them up. I had an employee that we requested go fragrance-free. About two years after they had given up using scented dryer sheets, they confessed to us that they had been so addicted to the smell that they would keep extra dryer sheets in their pockets and take them out and sniff them throughout the day. They shared that it was about six months before the cravings went away. This is not an isolated incident; the internet is full of stories of people who display similar behaviors with various laundry and fragranced products, and not just perfumes and colognes, but even bleach and cleaning products.

This same employee worked for us for more than ten years. They were amazed that after they became fragrance-free, they never got sick anymore. They would previously get colds, flu, sinus infections, sore throats, etc, multiple times a year. After they went fragrance-free and stopped using dryer sheets, they went more than nine years without getting sick. A woman I recently met and convinced to switch to a free and clear laundry detergent told me that within just a few weeks of using the fragrance-free products, her itchy skin problem disappeared. She had never even considered that her laundry detergent was causing her affliction.

I once worked in a small office. There were just two of us in the room most of the time: myself and another woman. She routinely wore perfume every day. I politely asked her not to wear it to work because I was having terrible headaches. She looked me in the eye and flat-out refused. I was flabbergasted;

did she not understand that she was making me sick? I tried to explain it to her and even got the boss involved, but she was adamant that I had no right to ask her to give it up. She said, "My husband gives me a bottle of this perfume for my birthday every year, and so I'm going to wear it whether you like it or not."

I was shocked. I'll never know how much of her position was due to an *addiction* to her perfume, or whether she just didn't like me, or both. The point is that people get all crazy about their fragrances, and their addictions will override their compassion more often than you would think.

If I ask you to stop wearing fragranced products, would your answer sound something equivalent to, "I can stop drinking anytime I want to; I just don't want to." How do you feel now that you know a chemist in a lab somewhere is manipulating you into making particular choices when it comes to your personal products?

What if you like to wear perfume but legally had to ask the permission of each person whose personal space it is going to infiltrate throughout the day—like asking, "Do you mind if I smoke?" It sounds ridiculous, but it illustrates the point that the people wearing fragrances in their laundry and personal products are basically deciding for the rest of us which toxins we will be unwillingly exposed to as we all go about our daily business.

Admittedly, I got kind of militant about this for a period of time. When I was well enough to go into restaurants again but still sick enough that the impact of secondhand fragrance would still be substantial, even through a short dinner, I went on a bit of a crusade. It's incredible to me now that any of my friends and family would still go anywhere with me after some of the scenes I caused in public places.

At one point, I even printed out little cards with a picture of a skunk with a little red circle and line across it on one side, and on the other side it advised the recipient to Google "Is fragrance toxic?" I would give these little cards to people in line in stores, random people in parking lots, doctor's offices, coffee shops, restaurants, you name it.

Sometimes I would point out to them that since it's considered bad manners to give negative feedback about the way someone smells, how is anyone to know that they smell bad, and wasn't that nice of me to tell them? I was just so incredibly frustrated and felt so helpless, and I wanted to fight back, but how? Did I really believe I was going to change anyone's behavior this way? Did I think anyone would look at that little card and say, "Wow, I had no idea, thanks for enlightening me!"

I came to the conclusion that when someone goes out in public wearing a fragrance, they are inviting interaction. After all, by choosing to influence the air others breathe with their personal preferences—something that could be seen as a form of assault—they are, in a way, inviting some level of response. I believe we all recognize this as an invitation, though society generally expects it to be a nonverbal interaction, especially if the response is not favorable. By expressing my reaction to the sensory experience being imposed on me without my permission, I was the one breaking the rules.

Perhaps this book is my new version of the little cards I gave out. I just keep thinking, "Maybe they just don't know." I have had the occasional success with acquaintances in sales, who quickly understood the implication that they were potentially alienating thirty percent of their potential clients just by wearing fragrance. If you are a salesperson or a realtor, for example, and work so hard and invest so much money to get leads and new clients, doesn't it just make sense to avoid offending thirty percent of those people and the potential income stream from them? They will never tell you they are choosing another business or another realtor because they don't like the way you smell. No one will ever say that to you (ok, except maybe me), and you'll always wonder why that customer or client chose a competitor over you when perhaps they just simply don't want to be around your secondhand fragrance.

This is an expensive disease. I remember sitting in a treatment room one day next to a woman who had been an environmental patient for considerably longer than me. She had been talking about how she needed to rotate her food so she didn't repeat eating any one thing within a four-day time frame, or she'd get really sick. She looked at me and said, "You know, this is not a disease for poor people."

At the time, I found her remark a bit off-putting and somewhat offensive, but it stuck with me. What she was really saying was that many people can't afford to treat this type of chronic disease or even have the resources to get a diagnosis—an unfortunate but very true reality.

For years, we paid for my treatment instead of putting money into a retirement fund. This was not optimal, but I was very grateful that at least it was an option for me. So many people get environmentally ill, and even if they are lucky enough to find a doctor who can recognize it and give a proper diagnosis, they can't afford to treat it.

That other patient was right. This is a very difficult disease, no matter who you are, but it helps to at least have the funds to treat it and manage the details. So many of these products with toxic ingredients are targeted and marketed directly at persons with low income; therefore a disproportionate number of environmentally ill people are struggling financially. How are they supposed to get a proper diagnosis, and treatment, and make all the necessary lifestyle changes?

Also, choosing organic and "safer" products tends to be more expensive. So, is a person without financial resources doomed to constantly expose themselves to toxins? Some people live in a food desert and have very limited options for produce, let alone organic. What are they supposed to do?

Laundry products don't just pollute the air around the people wearing the clothes; they pollute the air in the neighborhoods and cities where dryers are vented, and additionally create water pollution and affect our natural environment. *"Chemical emissions from residential dryer vents during use of fragranced laundry products" Air Quality, Atmosphere & Health, 2011 Anne C. Steinemann, Lisa G. Gallagher, Amy L. Davis, Ian C. MacGregor.*

But it's not just me or people like me you should be thinking about. These products are polluting the planet at an alarming rate. Everybody is so focused on the more obvious polluters, like cars, for example, that they are blissfully unaware of the fragrant elephant in the room. The February 2018 issue of Science magazine (vol 359, issue 6377) references studies that show while emissions from vehicles are on the decline, emissions from volatile chemical products (VCPs) are on the rise and now contribute equally, as in *one-half* of the emitted VOCs of the industrialized cities in the study. This should be front-page news! Our personal products, pesticides, inks, adhesives, cleaning products, etc., are causing air pollution *equal to the pollution from the cars we drive.* What will it take for people to notice?

If I can get triggered just from walking around my neighborhood or spending time in my own yard because of my neighbor's laundry choices, they are not doing themselves any favors either. Children do not need to wear clothing that is saturated with hormone disruptors. That seems so obvious. It breaks my heart when I see this. I know parents want the best for their children and would not intentionally harm them; they assume the products they buy in the grocery store are regulated for safety by our government, and that's just not always true.

CHAPTER 13

IS THE FDA ACTUALLY PROTECTING YOU?

The FDA website provides the following disclaimer: *Companies and individuals who manufacture or market cosmetics have a legal responsibility to ensure the safety of their products. Neither the law nor FDA regulations require specific tests to demonstrate the safety of individual products or ingredients. The law also does not require cosmetic companies to share their safety information with FDA.*"

In other words, the FDA actually allows the cosmetic industry to *self-regulate.*

Remember I had my tattoos lasered off because we found there was mercury in some of the ink? How could that be? Isn't tattoo ink regulated? Nope. The FDA does not regulate the ingredients of tattoo ink as it is considered a cosmetic. Again, from the FDA website: "*Although research is ongoing at the FDA and elsewhere, there are still a lot of questions about the long-term effects that may be caused by the pigments, other ingredients, and possible contaminants in tattoo inks. The FDA has received reports of bad reactions to tattoo inks right after tattooing and even years later. You also might become allergic to other products, such as hair dyes, if your tattoo contains p-phenylenediamene (PPD)."*

And also from the FDA in their article "Think Before You Ink: Tattoo Safety": *"Tattoo inks are colored liquid mixtures used to create body art. The inks contain pigments that are mixed with water and may contain a variety of other components, depending on the ink. Published research has reported that some inks contain pigments used in printer toner or in car paint. The FDA has not approved any pigments for injection into the skin for cosmetic purposes."*

Lastly, from the FDA in the same article: *"Then there's tattoo removal. We don't know the short- or long-term consequences of how pigments break down after laser treatment."*

I can personally attest to the statement about what happens when pigments break down after laser treatment. In addition to everything else presented about my tattoos, another thing happened that seems related. I started to develop a lump in one of my armpits several years ago that eventually got to be about the size of a large marble. Doctors examined it and could not determine what it was, so they advised me to have it surgically removed, which I did. Upon removal, the surgeon identified it as a mysterious sac full of dark or black unknown liquid, *like ink, he said.* It would appear, although this is unsubstantiated by testing, that when I was having my tattoos lasered off, my body was collecting the ink and storing it in my armpit.

Am I anti-tattoo? Not particularly; you do you. I am, however, pointing out another way that people erroneously make assumptions about the FDA protecting us, when in fact, the FDA points out the dangers of tattoos on their website and then basically says if you choose to get a tattoo, good luck, you are entirely on your own. Choose wisely.

Also, since we are deep-diving into the *facts* here, this is a big one:

From the FDA website on their position on fragrance in the article "Fragrances in Cosmetics": *"If a cosmetic is marketed on a retail basis to consumers, such as in stores, on the Internet, or person-to-person, it must have a list of ingredients. In most cases, each ingredient must be listed individually. But under U.S. regulations, fragrance and flavor ingredients can be listed simply as "fragrance" or "flavor."*

First of all, need I remind you that we have already seen that the FDA allows the fragrance industry to self-regulate? Therefore, you don't really know what is in your cosmetics when you see the word "fragrance" on the label. I'm assuming you read the labels. They could be putting anything into that fragrance, and they don't have to tell you. They won't tell you.

Secondly, that last sentence *implies* that the FDA considers *flavor* to be a fragrance, or rather, it categorizes them similarly. That's because, in many ways, flavor is a fragrance, not a food. The only actual *flavors* are salty, sweet, sour, bitter, and umami. Everything else is aroma. It's the aromas that define foods for us. If you were blindfolded and your nose was completely blocked, you would not be able to tell the difference between a lemon and a lime.

If you are buying pickle-flavored potato chips, let me assure you that, except in a few rare cases, no pickles were harmed in the creation of those chips. Their "pickle flavor" is a *chemical fragrance* that is added. Don't take my word for it; read the label. If it says nothing about pickles other than "natural flavorings," then you can thank Big Chemical for teaching chemists to use petroleum to *perfume* your chips so your sensory experience fools you into thinking you are eating pickle-flavored chips. And since petroleum is a natural product, the label can read "natural flavors," or "all-natural," or some other similar Bullshit.

From the website *ewg.org (a website whose mission is "To empower you with breakthrough research to make informed choices and live a healthy life in a healthy environment"*: *"How a food tastes is largely determined by the volatile chemicals in the food. Chemicals that give food a specific smell are extremely important because smell makes up 80 to 90 percent of the sense of taste. In processed food, this mixture of chemicals is called "flavor." The same mixture of chemicals would be called "fragrance" if it were found in cleaning products, perfumes or cosmetics. The difference between the two is small, and the companies that produce these secret mixtures are often exactly the same."*

According to the FDA, Title 21, Chapter I, Subchapter B: Food for Human Consumption: Part 101 Food Labeling; Subpart B: Specific Food Labeling Requirements: *"The term natural flavor or natural flavoring means the essential oil, oleoresin, essence or extractive, protein hydrolysate, distillate, or any product of roasting, heating or enzymolysis, which contains the flavoring constituents derived from a spice, fruit or fruit juice, vegetable or vegetable juice, edible yeast, herb, bark, bud, root, leaf or similar plant material, meat, seafood, poultry, eggs, dairy products, or fermentation products thereof, whose significant function in food is flavoring rather than nutritional."*

Again from *ewg.org: "These flavor mixtures often include amyl acetate, amyl butyrate, amyl valerate, ethyl butyrate, various aliphatic acid ester, ethyl acetate, ethyl valerate, ethyl isovalerate, ethyl pelargonate, vanillin, lemon essential oil, citral, citronellal,* *rose absolute, geraninol, orange essential oil, geranium essential oil, aldehyde C_{10}, ethyl heptanoate, acetaldehyde, aldehydes C_{14} and C_{16}, styralyl acetate, dimethyl benzyl carbinyl acetate, benzyl formate, phenyl ethyl isobutyrate, cinnamyl isovalerate, anise essential oil, esters of colophony and benzaldehyde and may contain terpenyl isovalerate, isopropyl isovalerate, citronellyl isovalerate, geranyl isovalerate, benzyl isovalerate, cinnamyl formate, isopropyl valerate, butyl valerate, methyl allyl butyrate and potentially the synthetic ingredients cyclohexyl acetate, allyl butyrate, allyl cyclohexylvalerate, allyl isovalerate and cyclohexyl butyrate."*

Do those ingredients sound "natural" to you? The natural or artificial emulsifiers, solvents, and preservatives in flavor mixtures are called "incidental additives." **That means the manufacturer does not have to disclose their presence on food labels.** Food manufacturers can use a natural solvent such as ethanol in their flavors, but the FDA also permits them to use synthetic solvents such as propylene glycol, *and they are not required to list it on the label as an ingredient.*

The same goes for so many processed foods that have a *fun* flavor or even those attractive flavored carbonated waters. You think you are making a healthy choice when you drink "lime-flavored" sparkling water instead of cola, but if the label says, "only carbonated water, naturally essenced," notice that it does not list "limes" as an ingredient. Again, no limes were harmed in the manufacturing of said lime-carbonated soda. It has been flavored or *fragranced* with a chemical that smells like lime, very possibly petroleum-based, and marketed as "all-natural." If you were unable to smell anything, it would have zero *flavor.*

The smell of our food is the nuance that makes us think it tastes a certain way, like the thing that makes an apple an apple and not a pear or a potato. The chemical companies understand this at a level most people do not suspect. Most of our processed food is designed to be addictive, with a quick punch of flavor that interacts with the pleasure center in our brain. Then, it is intended *not* to linger, so your brain screams for more. That is how they get you to eat an entire bag of neon orange cheesy poofs in one sitting.

When you see "natural flavors" on the label, you should ask yourself what that really means. Is this a "food" that has been chemically designed to manipulate your very thoughts and behavior? How often do you even read the labels of the packaged or processed food that you buy? And what are you looking for if you do read the labels?

Because I consider natural flavors to be quite unnatural, I generally have no desire to eat anything with "natural flavors," "all-natural," or "no artificial colors or flavors." If they are taking the trouble to put that on the label, it's because they are trying to trick us with Bullshit. Occasionally, I will make an exception and indulge in said neon orange cheesy poofs and think about my grandmother, but that is a very rare treat indeed.

Fragrances can be toxic. People who use fragrances are at higher risk for a multitude of afflictions, including cancer. According to: Cosmetics and Fragranced Products Pose High Risks for Breast Cancer and Other Illnesses by James W. Coleman, PhD., June 1, 2003: *"Beyond causing asthma, perfumes are also composed of substances recognized as neurotoxins, leading to a wide range of health issues. These include disorders affecting the central nervous system, reactions that trigger respiratory allergies, and irritations to the skin and eyes. Symptoms and conditions linked to perfume exposure encompass double vision, sneezing, nasal blockages, sinusitis, tinnitus, ear discomfort, dizziness, vertigo, coughing, bronchitis, breathing difficulties, trouble swallowing, anaphylactic reactions, headaches, seizures, exhaustion, confusion, disorientation, lack of coherence, short-term memory impairment, concentration problems, nausea, lethargy, anxiety, irritability, depression, mood fluctuations, restlessness, skin rashes, hives, eczema, facial redness, pain in muscles and joints, muscle weakness, irregular heartbeat, high blood pressure, and swollen lymph nodes, among others."*

This article deep dives into the connection between fragrances, personal products and cosmetics, and breast cancer. It goes on to indicate that perfumes are known to contain ingredients with addictive qualities and properties that induce a narcotic effect. The article shares that the scent of perfume can trigger immediate biochemical changes in the brain's pleasure center and that many perfumes include at least one narcotic component, with research indicating beauty products often possess additional addictive substances. This phenomenon could shed light on why some individuals frequently feel the need to "freshen up" multiple times throughout the day, essentially chasing another "high" in a manner reminiscent of traditional substance addiction.

As all of my environmental doctors informed me, these chemicals, carcinogens, and hormone disrupters compromise a person's immune system, making them more susceptible to illness. Babies, elderly persons, cancer patients, and ill people in general are especially affected by firsthand or also secondhand fragrances because their immune systems are not functioning at optimal levels. Hormone disruptors, including NPEs, which have been banned in the EU, are commonly found in many laundry products and are especially dangerous for pregnant women, babies, and teens. According to *ecos.com* (which promotes safe and sustainable cleaning products), studies show that NPEs can negatively affect fetal development, physical function, fertility, and may cause organ damage and/or cancer.

People instinctively know this, at least when it comes to babies because they will often choose alternate products for their babies rather than what they use for themselves. However, they overlook the fact that even if they are washing all of the baby's clothes and bedding with fragrance-free products, the baby is still being bombarded with chemicals by being in proximity to any adults using the fragranced products. Additionally, if a woman is breastfeeding the baby and she is using fragranced products, then the baby is really getting a full dose of chemicals.

A relative of mine once worked at a lab that processed a lot of photographs - analog film at the time, not digital. The workers there were exposed to photo-processing chemicals in the lab every day. One of her coworkers developed unusual skin growths on his face. After testing, it was discovered that these skin growths or lesions were primarily made up of the photo-processing chemicals he worked with daily. He had absorbed enough of these chemicals through his skin, and by breathing the fumes, that he developed growths partly composed of those very same chemicals.

When I was in Texas for treatment one year, I met a fellow patient who could not wear any clothes except organic, unbleached, undyed cotton. She revealed to me that before she was diagnosed with environmental illness, she had been living an everyday, healthy life when, suddenly, one of her hands started to turn blue. Not only that, but she could actually leave blue handprints on items that she touched. She went to her regular doctor, who sent her to a dermatologist. They could not figure it out, so they advised her to seek psychiatric help on the premise that she was doing this to gain attention. Eventually, she found her way to an environmental doctor who, through testing, was able to determine that *the blue dye coming out of her hands was originating from her blue jeans.* She was literally absorbing the blue dye from her jeans into her body and then processing it back out through the palms of her hands.

The skin is the largest organ of the body; that is a scientific fact. These anecdotes are meant to illustrate that we absolutely absorb chemicals through our skin, in addition to inhaling them with the air we breathe and ingesting them through the food we eat. Whatever we wash our clothes in, whatever is in our skin creams, makeup, shampoos, and other personal products, *is going to wind up inside our bodies as if we are eating it,* whether we choose to believe it or not.

The FDA does not oversee laundry products or other non-cosmetic fragranced products such as air fresheners or carpet fresheners. These, among other similar products, fall under the purview of the Consumer Product Safety Commission. The CPSC advises us not to eat the laundry pods because it's not safe to take those chemicals internally, but let me repeat – *when we put them on our bodies and in the air we breathe, we might as well be eating them because they still wind up inside of us just like food.* So why don't these products fall under the jurisdiction of the FDA? Not that I have any great love for the FDA or even any faith in their ability to actually regulate harmful chemicals, but at least then we'd officially be treating these products like food, *which our bodies are already doing.*

Some people go their whole lives oblivious to these exposures, seemingly with no ill effects. But how do you really know? Have you ever taken an aspirin for a headache, and it doesn't totally go away, and you wonder: would the headache be worse if you hadn't taken the aspirin? So maybe you didn't become chemically sensitive like me, or your hands are not turning the color of your jeans, but what if you had avoided fragrances and chemicals all your life? Maybe you would spend your entire life being super healthy, and perhaps you'd live longer, maybe another ten or twenty years, and all of them good years. How do you know what is in store for you next week? Is your toxic bucket almost full now, and is just one more dose of laundry or a new carpet going to be the thing to flip your switch?

Livestock are fed unnatural diets and live in crowded, unnatural conditions that all lend themselves to sickness and disease, thereby creating a dynamic where the animals in these feedlots are also consistently dosed with antibiotics and medicines, which also end up in our food.

The same is true for farmed fish, which is even more alarming because farmed fish are actually contaminating and destroying the local wild fish populations (newrootsinstitute.org). The very packaging of our food can contain a slew of unwanted chemicals and toxins. Americans, in general, choose to be blissfully unaware of where their food comes from, how it is grown, treated, packaged, and processed, and consequently, what they are actually eating.

We have been sold the idea that certain amounts of poisons or toxins are considered "safe" or "acceptable" in our food and in the products we put on our bodies and in our living spaces. The flaw here, well, one of the flaws, is that testing done on chemicals that determine how much exposure is safe is only done singularly. *(Silins I, Högberg J. Combined toxic exposures and human health: biomarkers of exposure and effect. Int J Environ Res Public Health. 2011 Mar;8(3):629-47. doi: 10.3390/ ijerph8030629. Epub 2011 Feb 24. PMID: 21556171; PMCID: PMC3083662.)* This study advises that the presence of multiple agents in our environment can alter the level of toxicity, either when these exposures occur together or one after another.

In cases of combined or mixed exposures, the resulting health impacts can be significantly greater than the sum of the effects of each component on its own. The requirement to account for a broader array of elements that influence the potential health impacts of combined exposures complicates the risk assessment procedure, making it more intricate than evaluating the risks associated with individual chemicals.

No one is considering what the consequences of a combined load of toxins are on our bodies until they get sick, and then it's too late. So maybe you can get away with the chemicals in your food, and maybe even also on your laundry, but the people who told you that those products are safe aren't considering the formaldehyde in the new carpet you just installed and the sunblock that you use on your skin every day, and the asbestos in your eye shadow and the mercury in your fillings.

Your personal toxin bucket is filling up whether you like it or not and whether you are aware of it or not. The only question remaining is, how much more can you put in your bucket before you end up like me?

Americans have been brainwashed into believing that the

world is a safe place. If it's on the shelf in the grocery store, whether it's food or cleaning products, you think it's safe. People assume that our government agencies are protecting them and their children and loved ones, but are they? Lobbyists have *way* too much power. The FDA states right on its website that it is allowing companies who create fragrances and cosmetics to self-regulate. Who is actually being protected here?

We wash our clothes with toxic chemicals. We douse ourselves in personal products that are loaded with toxic chemicals, some of which may be designed to manipulate us and affect our brains. We allow our crops to be genetically modified so they can be sprayed with toxic chemicals, which we then eat. We feed toxic chemicals and drugs to animals and let them live their lives in misery before we eat them with no thought to their sacrifices or the repercussions to the environment and, ultimately, ourselves. We let the insurance companies and the drug companies dictate how our doctors treat us. We are systematically destroying the planet and ourselves with our choices. What kind of world are we creating where all of this is okay? How many people are sick with chronic illnesses that could have been avoided? How long will it be before you or someone you love is sick like me?

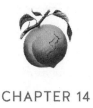

CHAPTER 14

DOCTORS

It has been my experience that if you have a hard-to-diagnose chronic illness, there is a high probability that you are screwed. My personal experience has been that the likelihood of getting a correct diagnosis *and* a successful treatment plan is low. By a successful treatment plan, I mean not spending the rest of your life dependent on drugs that have side effects as bad or worse than the symptoms you started with. I mean having treatment that identifies and treats the *root causes* of your affliction, not just the symptoms. I mean not being bullied or tricked into unnecessary surgery that will affect you for the rest of your life when you could have managed the problem with non-invasive treatment.

I *do* have great respect and admiration for doctors. But the system is failing the doctors first and, consequently, then failing all of us as well. Medical schools and their professors and lecturers have historically been dependent on funding from the pharmaceutical industry, thereby skewing the curriculum—-heavily weighing it in favor of a drug-based symptom-treating doctrine. This is a well-known and established fact, and as reported in the New York Times and Time magazine, even highly respected institutions like Harvard Medical School have been on the receiving end of millions of dollars from pharmaceutical companies. Although this dynamic has seen some change in very recent years, the damage is done, as the curricula are still very pro-drug treatment, and thousands of doctors have been released into the wild having been trained in this paradigm.

Additionally, insurance companies have *long* been dictating how much time doctors can spend with their patients and, at some level, how to diagnose and treat patients based on which expenses they are willing to cover. The result of all of this is an environment where average doctors do not have the training or the time to play detective for a patient with chronic illness presenting combinations of symptoms that seem to be unconnected to each other or any one specific cause. Nor do they have the flexibility to endorse treatment not covered by insurance for the typical patient. They have almost no choice other than to just prescribe drugs to manage the separate and seemingly unrelated symptoms.

Meanwhile, with the cause undetected and ignored, patients get sicker and require more drugs, more symptoms present themselves, including side effects from the drugs, and the cycle just repeats.

Of course doctors get frustrated trying to navigate these minefields, and I don't blame them. The system is designed to benefit the insurance and pharmaceutical companies, *not* the doctors and certainly not the patients. If the system were designed to truly benefit patients, the focus would be on *preventing* illness first and foremost. But that's not profitable for the big players who are running the show. By the way, did you know that insurance companies pay less for doctor visits and treatments than patients? Often, it is *substantially* less because the insurance companies get a bulk discount. I get the concept of buy more pay less, I really do, but it's outrageous that patients who have the wrong insurance or no insurance are very often forced to pay *more* than the going rate.

I will go to the doctor if I think it's appropriate. If I fracture a bone, cut myself, or sustain some other kind of mechanical injury, I want a doctor. If I have a heart attack, please call an ambulance for me. In general, if I need eyeglasses, I go to the eye doctor and have a fair expectation that my exam and consequent recommendations are appropriate and correct. If I have a sore throat that does not go away, I will seek testing and, if necessary, treatment for strep.

My PCP from the many years I suffered from chronic illness, is a kind, intelligent, and thoughtful doctor. I have always respected and admired her a great deal, and felt that she genuinely cared about my well-being. To her credit, when I started going to the environmental doctors, she was very supportive. In many ways, she provided excellent care for me over the years. But at some point, I clearly needed more than what she was able to provide, and it fell on me to figure it out for myself.

How did we get to a place where so many people are chronically ill and environmentally ill, and there are so few doctors who are trained to diagnose and deal with us? My issue isn't that all doctors aren't experts in environmental medicine. Obviously, every doctor is not an expert in every field. I don't want a podiatrist doing my breast lift. My issue is that environmental medicine is the unwanted bastard stepchild of modern medicine. Conventional doctors look the other way and pretend they don't exist instead of referring patients to them when things get murky. In addition, it is almost impossible to get insurance companies to pay for anything environmentally related.

I'm not anti-doctor, but I no longer think they know as much as we have been led to believe or what I used to think they knew. I recognize that there is massive pressure on them to have answers. No one wants to go to their doctor and be told, "I'm sorry, I have no idea what's really wrong with you, but we can experiment with different drug protocols to treat your symptoms and hope for the best."

I also recognize that in general, our doctors truly *want* to help and cure us, even when they don't know what to do. It has to be enormously frustrating to them when a chronically ill person walks through their door with a list of seemingly unrelated symptoms, and they don't have the time or the ability to figure it out.

So, our doctors do their best with the tools they have, which are too limited in the case of many chronic illnesses. How can our doctors possibly be expected to figure out what is wrong with us in the fifteen minutes or less that the insurance company has allotted for them to spend with each patient? The questionnaire I filled out for my environmental doctor was twenty-seven pages long. Most doctors don't have time for that kind of extensive review of your environmental history.

On top of that, they know that you likely want them to prescribe a pill to fix things. No one wants to be told, "Sorry, your mom should have handled her pregnancy more thoughtfully and not listened to her doctor, not taken DES, and then you should never have lived in a moldy house or worked at that factory or had all of that industrial carpet in an unventilated office, that's probably why you are sick, but we'll never really know. Here's a giant list of lifestyle changes you and everybody around you need to make; a lot of them are expensive, inconvenient, and painful. If you are lucky, you will eventually have some improvement."

If you walked into a doctor's office with mysterious pain, headaches, heart palpitations, hives, boils, angioedema, headaches, brain fog, and your hair falling out, and they said that to you, you'd probably walk out.

Also, I believe, they need to act like they know what they are doing, or the system would collapse. Many seem to have taken lessons from my Italian grandmother on how to say something with conviction so no one will question it. We have certain expectations from our doctors, and that affects how they treat and manage us, along with a whopping helping of interference from the insurance companies, misinformation and corporate greed supplied by the pharmaceutical companies, and lack of education in medical school on environmental and alternative medicine.

I have friends who are doctors, and I hope like hell that if they read this book, they will continue to be my friends. I hope and imagine that they might not disagree with everything I have to say. We, the patients, are part of the problem because we don't want to be told any inconvenient truths; we just want a pill to solve everything, myself included. But there is no magic elixir, and it's a long, hard road to recognizing that. As long as the typical medical school curriculum ignores the fact that our environment is a critical factor in our health and well-being and is often a major factor in the origins of our diseases, then we can't expect our doctors to be something other than what they have been trained to be.

Chiropractors saved my life. I believe this to be an absolute fact. After I was injured at the factory, I genuinely believe that if I had let one of those surgeons operate on me, I would have endured a lifetime of pain and more surgeries, eventually leading to me being completely incapacitated and always in pain. Not once did any of my doctors advise me to see a chiropractor, especially before submitting to surgery.

However, a chiropractor was able to provide me with a diagnosis and treatment that did not include drugs or surgery and successfully started me on a path to regain life. Chiropractors have been there for me ever since, keeping those same problems in check.

How is it possible that no doctor ever sent me to a chiropractor? In fact, some people I know in conventional medicine have frowned upon my chiropractic treatment despite the excellent non-surgical, non-invasive, positive, and life-changing results I have experienced for decades. How dare you!

By the way, it was also a chiropractor who put me on a weight loss program that actually worked for me at age fifty-something, when all other doctors had basically said to me, "You should lose weight, exercise, and don't eat cake; good luck."

No doctor ever advised me to get acupuncture either. Yet, my acupuncturist instantly knew what was wrong with me; I just wasn't ready to hear it. I still wanted a magic pill back when I first went to her. I still believed doctors knew the answers, and I still trusted them to heal me at the time. I wasn't open to what she told me, and unfortunately, it took years for me to get to a place where I accepted what she had said from the beginning and then allowed her to be part of my healing process.

Despite my experiences with orthopedic surgeons back in

my factory days, I do think many surgeons are talented and brilliant and have a lot to offer. They save and improve lives every single day. But that doesn't mean that every surgery being sold to a patient is necessary or even helpful.

I think neurologists have their place, but they did not help my mother, nor, in my opinion, did they truly participate in the fieldwork of researching the root cause of her Alzheimer's, although they claimed to do exactly that. Don't get me wrong, they were kind to her and dutifully prescribed the appropriate meds to slow down the disease. But they never once asked even one question about her environmental history, diet, or living situation.

How can you research an *environmental* disease without chronicling the *environmental* history of your patients to create a database that can correlate common factors and exposures? Why aren't doctors required to participate in something like that? Why are they not incentivized to prevent disease in the first place rather than just treat it after it's too late? I'm calling Bullshit on that.

Well, it's naive to think that if it's on the grocery store shelf or my doctor can prescribe it to me, it's safe. It's time we recognized that it's up to *us* to practice preventative medicine ourselves, not wait to get sick and then hope for a cure or wait for our doctors to tell us what to do.

Our heads have been in the sand for too long. We've looked the other way while these corporations have systematically been destroying our health and our planet. I've been hard on doctors, but they are not the enemy. They are as much the victims as the rest of us, with Big Pharma and Big Chemical holding all the cards and influencing the path of Western medicine for decades.

The only way out of this is for us first to recognize what is happening and then stop *mindlessly* giving our power away to the people we have long been brainwashed into trusting, such as our doctors and our politicians.

It's time to become our own advocates. Open our eyes and look around. Stop assuming that everyone else knows what's best for you and your family and that anyone else is acting in your best interest. Expect and demand to be part of your medical process and be a steward of your own records. Look for correlations yourself. Make good and healthy choices.

Vote with your wallet. Money always talks in the end. That's how we got here in the first place. Money has been greasing the palms of the people who make the decisions for the masses forever, but we are *not* helpless. We can fight back by simply choosing not to buy products that make us sick. It really is just that simple.

CHAPTER 15

WHERE AM I NOW?

So what is it, or what was it? Was it a brain injury from my fall in the restaurant and/or toxic overload from all my early exposures to mold and industrial and factory chemicals? Was the DES and my mom's drinking and smoking during pregnancy a factor? Or is it a combination of all those things or even something else entirely? I have asked myself those same questions repeatedly. The truth is, I still don't really know and probably never will. What's important now, is to recognize what I have learned along the way.

I strive to lead a healthy lifestyle and think of myself as a healthy person now. I think about what I put in or on my body, not just physically but also mentally and emotionally. I'm not always successful, but it's in my awareness now, so I am always trying. I also try to make exercise an important part of my life, although admittedly, I have stumbled recently. But I don't beat myself up over it. I'm less critical of myself these days and realize life is meant to be enjoyed.

After my mom died, we sold our business and our house, and then Dene, our dog Sprout, and I moved into our Airstream trailer full-time. We drove around the country for a while, trying to decide where we wanted to live next. Ultimately, we ended up in New Mexico, but it wasn't always easy getting here. As mentioned, RV living has challenges, especially full-time with no washing machine! I think Dene could have kept going in the camper indefinitely, but Sprout and I grew tired of it. We found a house that we love in a great neighborhood with plenty of space and friendly people. Our new home has tile floors and is easy to air out as needed.

I have learned to manage my exposures in a way that allows me to live a reasonably normal life most of the time. I have come to accept certain limitations but am also able to embrace new opportunities. I hold out hope for the day when I can travel with complete freedom and don't have to make annoying demands of friends and family, but I don't obsess over it anymore.

Laundry products are still the bane of my existence, which continues to limit my ability to travel and socialize, but I'm working on it. Because I manage my exposures so well most of the time, when I do have them, my recovery is usually pretty quick. If I want to take a plane somewhere (I still need an excellent reason), I won't enjoy it and in fact dread it, but I can do it. Hotels and other lodgings are still problematic, but I'm working on solving that problem for all of us.

I read the label on almost every single thing I purchase and try to make good choices. I am still vegetarian one hundred percent of the time and do not expect to ever eat meat again intentionally. At home, we rarely have eggs or dairy. When we eat out, we allow ourselves dairy and the occasional egg. I strive to shop for organic, non-GMO, and non-processed foods. At home, we still avoid canola oil, and most of the time, we eat gluten-free. I can't remember the last time I had heart arrhythmia or chest pain.

Our new house has a pizza oven, which accounts for a large percentage of any gluten or dairy we eat at home, but it's still very minimal. I've been experimenting with the excellent sourdough bread from the local farmer's market. There is a lot of chatter out there about how people who are sensitive to gluten can eat sourdough bread without any ill effects. So far I seem to be getting away with it a couple of times a week, something I never thought would happen.

When we were traveling full time, we got out of the habit of exercising regularly, so between that, the local wineries, and the cheese, I gained some weight when we settled into our new house. I've been working on it though, and am finally back to where I was when we left Massachusetts.

I am much kinder to myself about my weight these days and recognize that my weight does not dictate who I am any more than my chemical sensitivity does. I am so much more than numbers on a scale or a collection of symptoms. I just want to be healthy, feel good, and start every day knowing good things will happen because they *will* if I look for them and align myself with that reality.

I generally avoid people who aren't fragrance-free, especially people who use scented laundry. I rarely try to get people to change anymore because I recognize they don't want to for many reasons. I'm done crusading at a personal level. I get too involved and emotional. I only make the effort now when I see a real benefit to having a specific person in my life.

We have a saltwater pool at our new home. It's fantastic because I can swim in it without all the problems of chlorine exposure. I've learned to be careful about who we invite to swim because the pool can get contaminated with laundry products and sunblock. At one point last year, I thought we might have to drain the pool because some people who were covered in super-fragranced laundry products swam in it. Fortunately, over a period of several weeks, it got filtered out on its own, but it sure did throw me for a loop for a hot minute.

So, I still get blindsided now and then. Partly because I'm doing so much better, I'm a little too cavalier about my abilities sometimes. Even though I feel like I've got this thing figured out and managed, weird stuff still sneaks up on me and catches me off guard.

So, am I better? Am I healed, cured? Yes and no. Is that the end of the story? As I write this today, I am fifty-nine years old. I was forty-five when I walked into Dr. L's office without a clue. My journey has been painful, difficult, sometimes seemingly hopeless, but ultimately profound and rewarding. No, I am not precisely "cured," but I am better.

In many ways, you could say that I am healed, certainly in my heart and soul, and that is what really makes my life worth living now. I have learned how to choose to be happy, and so I am happy. I have had a fundamental shift in how I view the world and myself, bringing me personal peace and happiness. Every minute is not perfect, and most likely will never be, but I accept that and am ok with it.

The magic here is that I am helping not only my own health with my choices but also the planet. Isn't it interesting that the earth's health is tied so directly to the choices we make for our *own* health? Because I don't eat meat, I have one-fourth of the environmental impact of someone who does eat meat. I'm not suggesting that everyone suddenly needs to become plant-based, although that would be great. But I am saying that our choices have consequences, and I am pleased to be making much more informed choices these days. I'm taking control of my health and, consequently, my impact on the world we all live in and, therefore all of the beings who live in it, including you. You're welcome.

So, I'm doing great, thanks for asking. I now think of myself as happy, healthy, and strong. And so it is true. Today is a great day!

P.S. I'm still trying to grow the elusive perfect tomato.

AFTERWORD

It is my heartfelt desire that this book will accomplish several things. I want other chronically ill people to have hope and know that there is a light at the end of the tunnel. I want them to believe in themselves, trust what they know about their bodies, and take their power back—demand to have a voice in their treatment and question everything. Perhaps more importantly, know that you can *choose* happiness even when the struggle for good health seems hopeless.

I don't have all the answers, certainly not for myself, much less anyone else. But I want to share what I have learned because it was a long, painful, and expensive road to get where I am now. I was fortunate to figure some of this out before it got worse. I know there are plenty of people out there who could be helped by making some of the same changes that I did and possibly avoid or reduce suffering because of it. By sharing my story, and the lessons I have learned, just maybe, I can make a difference.

I would ask people to examine the products they use every day and consider how those products are affecting not just themselves but everybody else they come into contact with and the world we all live in. Perhaps you think you are bullet-proof and none of this concerns you, or you don't care about

EVERYTHING IS *NOT* PEACHEY

the stranger sitting nearby in a restaurant or beside you on an airplane. But what about the people or pets you do care about? Elderly, babies, cancer patients, chronically ill people - none of them can afford to have their immune systems work any harder than they already are. By default, if you make better choices for the people you love, you will also be making better choices for yourself and our planet, which will better serve you and the people you love.

I would humbly request that people try to buy organic whenever possible. As previously mentioned, we vote with our wallets. And I know very well that sometimes the conventional tomatoes or potatoes look so much prettier than the organic ones, but remember, it's a lie, and in the end, one of them is filling that invisible bucket full of toxins, and the other is not. Whenever I've seen news stories about organic versus conventional vegetables, the focus is always on studies that show organic vegetables are not necessarily more *nutritional* than conventional vegetables. This is just a distraction, a misdirection from the real problem. We need to support the organic movement whenever possible if we want to save ourselves and our planet.

Remember, thoughts matter. When I catch myself having monkey-brain, obsessing over something negative, I consciously halt and replace those thoughts with a positive mantra instead, something like: "I am happy, healthy, and strong..." I add all kinds of positive affirmations to the end of that and repeat it several times, and suddenly, I am free of whatever negative thoughts I might have been stuck in. Nightbirde was right to tell the world, "We can't wait for everything to be perfect to choose to be happy." I now choose happiness, and I hope you will too. No matter how bad things are, it's worse when you wallow in it and better when you choose happiness.

Please be kind to your animals and all animals. Be grateful when they provide you with food or other products. Be thoughtful about the chemicals we expose them to and how they are treated when they are part of our food chain. They all deserve our respect, kindness, and gratitude. Remember that if you think your dryer sheets have a strong smell, you can't even begin to imagine what it's like for your dog to be assaulted with it.

A fragrance-free trend is gaining momentum, and it is important to me to promote and encourage that. I am endeavoring to educate people and make that not just a trend but mainstream. I would love to see hotels and Airbnbs jump on that bandwagon. There *are* a few out there, but not nearly enough, not even close. I'd like to see fragrance or sensitivity ratings for hotels and rentals right next to cleanliness and cost on mainstream review platforms.

That's why I've created the website www.peacheyreport. com—a dedicated platform for people with allergies and sensitivities, as well as vegans and vegetarians, offering a directory of places and products that cater to our needs. I hope that, together, we can build a comprehensive resource that supports a growing community. If we can't change the industry overnight, we can still make a difference by highlighting and supporting businesses that prioritize our health and needs. I'm working hard to launch it soon with all the information I've gathered, and I encourage you to join me in making this resource as valuable as possible for everyone who needs it.

So, let's begin a new journey together. Let's rebuild our health, our state of mind, and the world around us.

Thank you for letting me share my story with you.

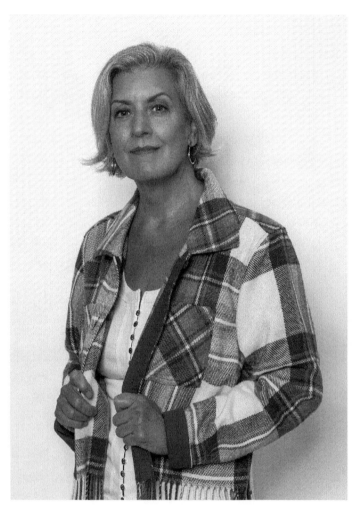

The author in summer of 2024.

RESOURCES

Useful Websites:

awionline.org
Animal rights website

chem-tox.com
Information on the effects of chemicals and pesticides

clearya.com
App for shopping non-toxic products

congress.gov/bill/117th-congress/house-bill/5538/text
Cosmetic Fragrance and Flavor Ingredient
Right to Know Act of 2021

dldewey.com/perfume.htm
Information on the effects of chemicals,
fragrances and pesticides

ewg.org/skindeep
A guide to safer personal products

invisibledisabilities.org
Resources for people with invisible disabilities

maskedcanaries.wordpress.com
Useful information and resources for environmentally ill people

newrootsinstitute.org
Animal rights and info about how
factory farming affects humans also

onegreenplanet.org
Miscellaneous resources for health
animal welfare, and the environment

PeacheyReport.com
Reviews and Product Recommendations
for people with allergies and sensitivities

safecosmetics.org
A program of Breast Cancer Prevention Partners (BCPP), a national
science-based advocacy organization working to prevent breast cancer
by eliminating environmental exposures linked to the disease.

silentspring.org
Data on the environment and its effect on women's health

wickedkitchen.com
Outstanding plant based recipes

womensvoices.org
Women's Voices for the Earth: drives action towards a future
free from the impacts of toxic chemicals rooted in gender
justice alongside those historically and presently ignored by
the environmental health movement by leveraging an intersec-
tional solidarity approach based on our expertise in research,
advocacy and organizing.

ALSO BY LISA PEACHEY

Bobarino's Word Search Puzzle Book:
Puzzles Inspired by Crazy Shit My Dad Says...

The puzzles are inspired by my dad, who you may recall has a unique cavalier perspective on certain things. This is the story of my dad, told in 100 unique word search puzzles.

• • •

ALSO BY LISA PEACHEY AND CO-AUTHORED BY CAROL ELIZABETH LONG:

369 Manifest Journal:
A Phase I Creative Studio From Miley,
Your Multidimensional Guide

*Now in Special Edition with Bonus Material, which shares the original transcripts of our first two sessions with Miley through communicator Carol Elizabeth Long

ABOUT THE AUTHOR

Lisa Peachey happily lives in New Mexico with her husband, Dene, their dogs, Sprout, Lewis, and Clark, along with Sprout's three fancy goldfish.

Lisa is always looking for new ways to share her experiences and make the world a better place. With that in mind, she manages **PeacheyReport.com**.

Lisa created this website as a resource for people with allergies and sensitivities where she features a comprehensive database of businesses and products that she endorses for people with allergies and sensitivities.

On the website, you can find hotels that use fragrance-free laundry products and/or have no carpet in the rooms, restaurants with excellent gluten-free or allergy-friendly menus, and restaurants with good vegan or vegetarian options. It also has links to products, such as fragrance-free and cruelty-free makeup that is also really good, or where to buy Lisa's favorite organic mattress.

Finally, Lisa also encourages you to join in by participating in the community.

If you have questions for Lisa about this book or have a recommendation that is relevant to people with allergies and sensitivities, or vegans/vegetarians, you can contact Lisa through the website.

Or, if you prefer, you can connect via social media. Just look for Peachey Report on Facebook, Instagram, X, and maybe TikTok.

Thank you so much for taking the time to read *Everything is Not Peachey*. Your support means the world to me. I would truly appreciate it if you could share your thoughts by leaving a review. Your feedback not only helps me as an author, but it also helps other readers discover the book and understand how it might resonate with them.

ACKNOWLEDGEMENTS

Photo of Mom and Dad on the beach
taken by Orlando Wedding Pix

Photos of Lisa
by Tina Dwyer Photography

Made in United States
Orlando, FL
30 October 2024

53292938R00112